IMAGES
of America

Medical Society of Erie County

On the Cover: Pictured here is an ambulance around the turn of the 20th century during the Pan-American Exposition. (Courtesy of the Medical Society of Erie County.)

IMAGES
of America

Medical Society of Erie County

Stacey Watt, MD, MBA, FASA and
Aimana ElBahtity, Esq.
Foreword by Robert S. Armstrong, MD, FACS

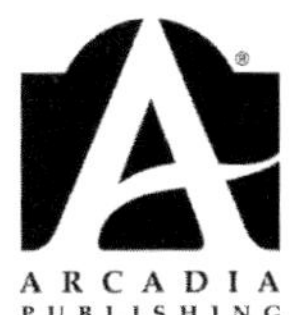

ISBN 978-1-4671-0747-1

Published by Arcadia Publishing
Charleston, South Carolina

Printed in the United States of America

Library of Congress Control Number: 2021942489

For all general information, please contact Arcadia Publishing:
Telephone 843-853-2070
Fax 843-853-0044
E-mail sales@arcadiapublishing.com
For customer service and orders:
Toll-Free 1-888-313-2665

Visit us on the Internet at www.arcadiapublishing.com

Dedicated to the physicians, past and present,
of the Medical Society of Erie County, New York,
in appreciation of their dedicated service in medicine, both
historically and today during these unprecedented times.

Contents

Foreword

As the Medical Society of the County of Erie (or Medical Society of Erie County) celebrates its 200th anniversary, we wanted to take this opportunity to look back at the rich history of our region and the vital role medicine has played in it. Buffalo, New York, and its surrounding communities have influenced medical care and innovation in more ways than people realize. Often thought of only for its snowfall, most people would never expect to discover that Buffalo was where the first woman graduated from medical school or that Jamestown was home to the first phenylketonuria (PKU) screening test.

From the Medical Society's inception on September 21, 1821, to today, our physician members have selflessly and skillfully served the western New York region. We are proud of our long tradition and commitment to medical care in this community. In fact, the Medical Society of the County of Erie is the second oldest medical society in the United States.

Today, the Medical Society seeks to maintain ethical standards in the physician community, educate the public on health matters, and help ensure the availability of high-quality health care for the citizens of Erie County.

We hope you enjoy this collection of inspiring stories and interesting highlights of medicine in Erie County. The contributions of the remarkable men and women who have gone before us in this field spur us all on. We are proud to help document this heritage.

—Robert S. Armstrong, MD, FACS
200th President, Medical Society of the County of Erie

Acknowledgments

Stacey Watt, MD, authored the chapter introductions, and Aimana ElBahtity, Esq., authored the photograph captions.

For the research that went into obtaining images for this book, the authors would like to thank Cynthia VanNess, MLS, director of Library and Archives, Buffalo History Museum; Jessica Hollister, MLIS, assistant librarian, University Archives, University at Buffalo; and Tineke Hall for her extensive research and administrative work.

We are also very appreciative of the work of Jane S. Woodward, author of *Men of Medicine in Erie County 1821–1971*, which was published in 1971 to honor the 150th anniversary of the Medical Society of the County of Erie. We now publish this book to honor the Medical Society's marking of its 200th anniversary.

Unless otherwise noted, all images appear courtesy of the Medical Society of the County of Erie.

Please note: In 1962, the University of Buffalo merged with the State University of New York and its name was changed to State University of New York at Buffalo, also referred to as the University at Buffalo (UB) or SUNY Buffalo. In addition, the School of Medicine's name changed to the Jacobs School of Medicine and Biomedical Sciences. All variations of the university and medical school names are used in this text where appropriate.

INTRODUCTION

The War of 1812 brought upheaval within our nation and set in motion the wheels of change. The changes were felt acutely within Buffalo as neighbors clung together while the city was burned to the ground. As war raged along the American-Canadian border, wreaking havoc on the border towns, there was a strong desire on both sides to gain the upper hand before the looming winter cold arrived. As the snow began to fall, the British forces were still reeling from a recent defeat in York (present-day Toronto). To quench their thirst for revenge, the British troops charged over the border in the predawn hours of December 19, 1813, attacking Fort Niagara. After the fort was destroyed, the offensive continued as the nearby villages of Lewiston and Youngstown were attacked. Although their victory dealt a blow to American forces, it was not enough to satisfy British lieutenant general Gordon Drummond.

The newly settled, small trading communities of Black Rock and Buffalo were next to bear attacks from the north. On December 30, shortly after midnight, British forces again crossed the border and attacked these fledgling cities. The soldiers destroyed everything in their path—homes, businesses, and gathering places. Torches were lit and hurled onto the wooden structures, setting them ablaze. The flames burned most of Buffalo to the ground, with only 100 or so buildings still standing. But the city would not be lost. Within a week of the attack, the residents began to rebuild, and Buffalo slowly resumed its rise into the chapters of our country's history.

The spirit of this small city would not be denied. As Buffalo began to grow, an opportunity of national significance was delivered to the area in the form of the Erie Canal. The canal began construction in 1817 and was completed in 1825. It stretched over 363 miles from Albany to Buffalo, making it the longest artificial waterway in North America. The building of the canal put New York on a path to become a leader in industry and an economic powerhouse. The waterway not only connected industry, but created a conduit for innovation, wealth, and immigration. The Erie Canal, or "Gateway to the West" as it was commonly called, was responsible for propelling Buffalo's growth into the 1900s.

As Erie County was experiencing a boom of growth and development, an organization within this up-and-coming region of the United States was also starting its journey. The Medical Society of the County of Erie was founded in September 1821. The society began as a means of fulfilling a requirement of New York state law, since all physicians within the state were required to belong to a local medical society.

The law of the time also gave medical societies the legal authority to judge the fitness of physicians engaging in medical practice as well as the ability to set clinical, educational, and ethical standards of the medical practice.

The 24 charter members of the Medical Society of the County of Erie met on September 21, 1821, in the home of R.M. Pomeroy at Main and Seneca Streets within the village of Buffalo. At this inaugural meeting, Cyrenius Chapin, MD, a veteran of the War of 1812, was elected the society's first president.

While Buffalo continued its rise into the national spotlight, physicians and lawyers within the county recognized the need to foster the development of its medical community. The University of Buffalo School of Medicine was founded in 1846. Medical classes began on February 24, 1847, with an enrollment of 66 students as medicine and society advanced.

Erie County's connection to innovation was not limited. The county has been home to many groundbreaking scientists who have changed the face of medicine. Carl Ferdinand Cori won the Nobel Prize in Physiology or Medicine in 1947 for his work on the Cori cycle of metabolism, which outlined how lactic acid forms when we exercise and is converted into glycogen within the liver. Born in Prague, Cori moved to Buffalo in 1922 to continue his research on metabolic pathways and then moved on to Washington University in St. Louis.

Sir John Carew Eccles also won a Nobel Prize in Medicine in 1963 for his work on the study of higher brain functions. He shared the award with Alan Hodgkin and Andrew Huxley for discovering the mechanism for chemical communication between neurons across nerve cell junctions. Thanks to his discovery, scientists were better able to understand the brain and its intricate workings.

As medical education and innovation flourished within Erie County, the city of Buffalo continued its explosive industrial growth. The New York Central Railroad connected the Great Lakes and mid-Atlantic regions of the United States. The railroad was established in 1853 and worked to consolidate smaller existing railroads, easing the path of transit across the growing country. The New York Central began work on the Buffalo Terminal in 1925, further positioning Buffalo to become one of the nation's economic powerhouses.

As railroads were built, waterways flourished, and Buffalo bustled with energy and growth. The city also became home to innovators who changed how we practice the art of medicine. Erie County was the home of Wilson Greatbatch and Dr. William Chardack. Greatbatch, an electrical engineer and inventor, worked alongside Dr. Chardack, chief of surgery at the Buffalo Veterans Affairs Hospital. Together, they developed the first successful human cardiac pacemaker, which was implanted on June 6, 1960. The city was also home to Dr. Jack Lippes, an obstetrician-gynecologist who designed an intrauterine device (IUD) in the form of a plastic double-S loop that reduced the incidence of pregnancy. The Lippes Loop was first sold in 1962 and quickly became the most widely prescribed IUD in the nation. Another innovator was Dr. Robert Guthrie, who devoted his medical career to researching the prevention of developmental disabilities, setting out to produce a simple screening tool for infants. His background as a professor of microbiology and pediatrics helped him to develop a screening test for phenylketonuria (PKU). This genetic disorder results in the body's inability to break down amino acids and results in mental and physical disabilities in children. The first screening took place in 1961 in Jamestown, and Guthrie's blood spot–testing method spread, leading the charge for the development of multiple newborn screening tests that are still in use today.

In 1897, the Pan-American Exposition Company was looking for a place to hold its exposition. Buffalo was selected for this prestigious honor because of its size and location. It was the eighth-largest city in the nation at the time and boasted extensive railway connections, which made travel to and from the exposition much easier. The educational exhibits would showcase the latest and greatest advancements of technology, innovation, and electricity. A highlight of the event was the electric lighting that utilized hydroelectric power generated by the nearby Niagara Falls. The exposition created a never-before-seen event filled with light bulbs and a prominent electric tower, which lit the night sky. The Pan-American Exposition launched Buffalo into the national spotlight not only for the innovation displayed on the midway, but also for the assassination of Pres. William McKinley.

Erie County's connection to the US presidency began on September 6, 1901. While greeting guests of the Pan-American Exposition at the Temple of Music, President McKinley was shot twice. He was immediately taken to the exposition's hospital, where he was operated on by a number of prominent surgeons from the Erie County community, including Dr. Roswell Park. The president was taken home to recover, but eventually died on September 14 due to infection and gangrene that resulted from his gunshot wounds. Knowledge of the passing of President McKinley reached Vice Pres. Theodore Roosevelt while he was vacationing nearby in the Adirondacks. Arriving by train, Roosevelt took the presidential oath of office in the home of Ainsley Wilcox.

William Howard Taft was another president who visited Erie County. His arrival on April 30, 1910, to speak at a chamber of commerce dinner also included a visit with many community leaders. Presidents Harry Truman, Herbert Hoover, Dwight Eisenhower, John Kennedy, Lyndon Johnson, Gerald Ford, Jimmy Carter, Ronald Reagan, Bill Clinton, George H. Bush, George W. Bush, Barack Obama, and Donald Trump also made visits to Buffalo to network and preside over community celebrations.

Erie County had been a scene of tremendous growth and prosperity, but the summer of 1967 saw a terrible turn when race riots shook the nation. The summer, also called the "long hot summer," saw the eruption of 159 race riots in many cities, including Buffalo. One riot occurred on the east side of Buffalo from June 26 to July 1 when a small group of teenagers broke into cars and shattered store windows. Two hundred riot-ready police officers were summoned to stem the unrest, but a violent encounter resulted in a shutdown of the city by its leaders.

In contrast to the heat that set the city ablaze, Erie County is primarily known for snowfall and frigid temperatures. No other event has defined the city for its climate more than the Blizzard of 1977. The storm began on January 28 with wind gusts peaking at 69 miles per hour and a record snowfall as high as 100 inches in some areas around the city. While new snow was a factor, much of the snow was actually blown in from piles resting on top of the frozen Lake Erie. Gusting winds carried the snow into drifts of 30 to 40 feet high. Snowmobiles became the primary means of transportation, carrying medical workers to and from hospitals to care for the many injured citizens.

The medical history of Erie County again came to center stage in 2001 when the Buffalo Niagara Medical Campus (BNMC) was founded. The BNMC now includes over seven institutions, including the Roswell Park Cancer Institute, Buffalo General Hospital, and the University at Buffalo School of Medicine. The medical campus encompasses 6.5 million square feet and supports clinic, research, education, and support space. This organization has been a shining example of the collaborative environment of the city and the campus as it continues to grow.

The Medical Society of the County of Erie has played a vital role in the journey of this region. Whether caring for a president shot while celebrating our city or racing through impassable snow-laden streets on snowmobiles to ensure our citizens received lifesaving care, our medical society has been sewn into the fabric of our community and will continue to be a shining example of the very best we have to offer.

One

The Burning of Our City

The frigid cold winter of 1813 brought more than a continuation of the War of 1812, it brought with it the events that would set into motion the destruction of Buffalo. In retaliation for the destruction of Niagara on the Lake by American forces, British troops and their Native American allies captured Buffalo, and on December 31, 1813, after the battle was over, burned the city to the ground.

In August 1814, the city was again under attack from British forces, but this time they were defeated by a small force of American riflemen under Maj. Lodwick Morgan at the Battle of Conjocta Creek. At the time of the retreat, Buffalo only had a few remaining structures that survived the chaos, but by 1815, the city had rebuilt from the ashes.

Rebuilding after the Battle of Buffalo marked the start of a series of developments that would propel Buffalo into the national spotlight. The year 1825 marked the completion of the Erie Canal, with Buffalo as a port of call for settlers on their journey westward. The opening of the waterway put Buffalo in a position to control trade flowing into and out of the nation's expanding interior. New settlements sent crops east toward New York City, while consumer goods flowed west to the new settlers through the canal.

The construction of the Erie Canal brought not only commerce to Buffalo, but a surge in the population of the Queen City. The population boom saw the city doubling in size in the mid-1800s, and by 1855, almost two thirds of the city's population were foreign-born immigrants.

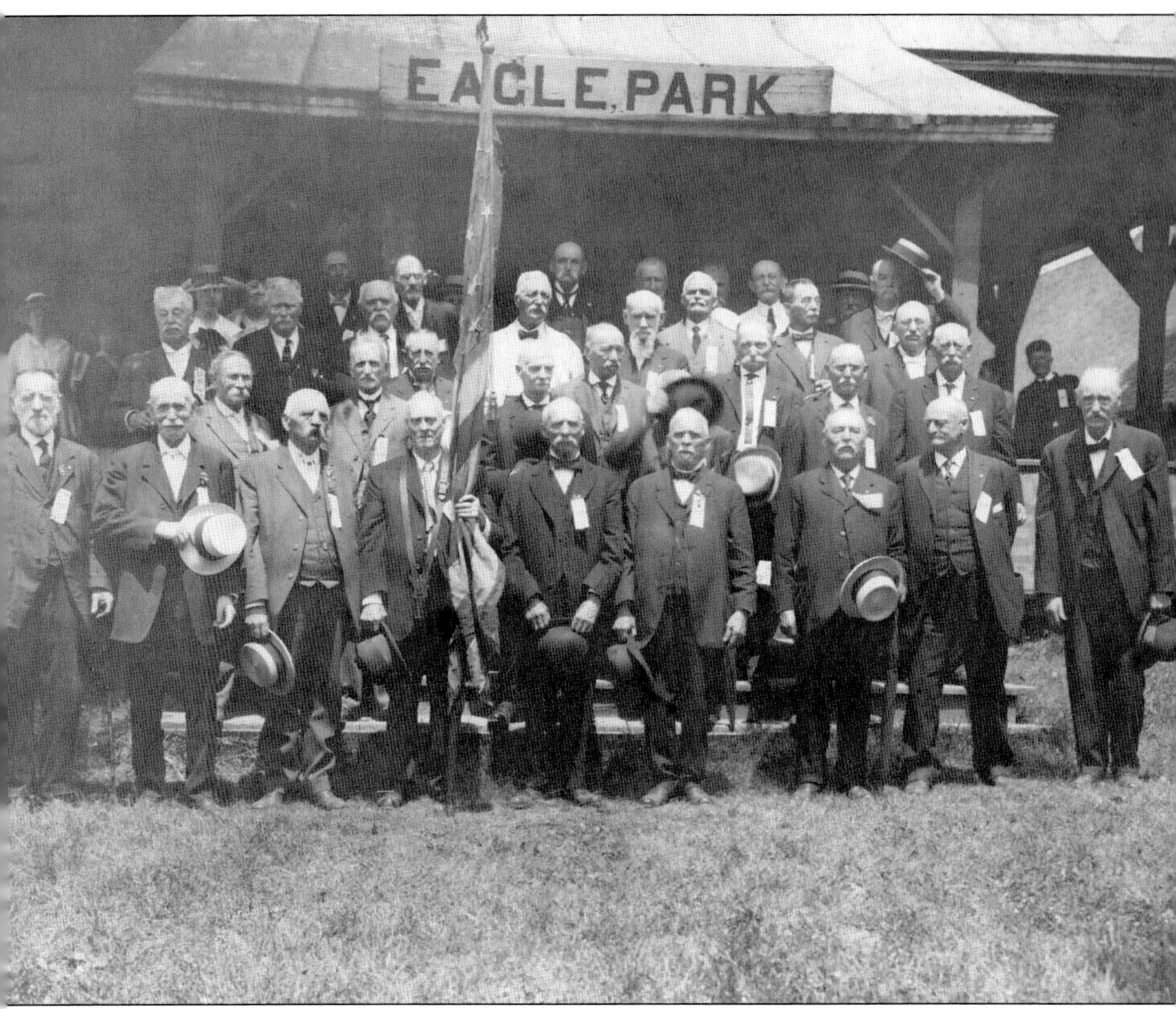

Seen here is a reunion of the men who served in the 21st Regiment during the Civil War. Eagle Park is along the West River in Grand Island, New York. Dr. Frank Hamilton, one of the founders of the university's School of Medicine, served as a surgeon in the Civil War. (Courtesy of the Buffalo History Museum, General Photograph Collection, Military–Civil War–Regiments.)

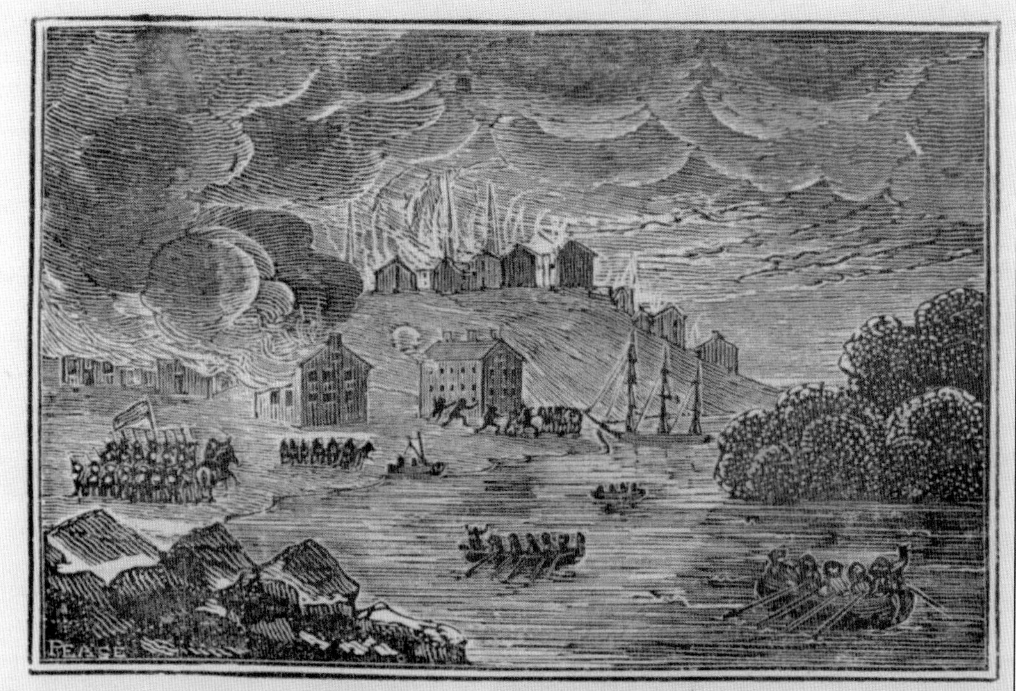

This 1813 illustration depicts the burning of the city of Buffalo by the British during the War of 1812. The Medical Society of Erie County's founder and its first physician-president, Cyrenius Chapin, was captured by the British while serving as a major. Following his release from Montreal, Dr. Chapin returned to Buffalo where he founded the Medical Society on September 1, 1821. (Courtesy of the Buffalo History Museum, General Photograph Collection, Buffalo Views.)

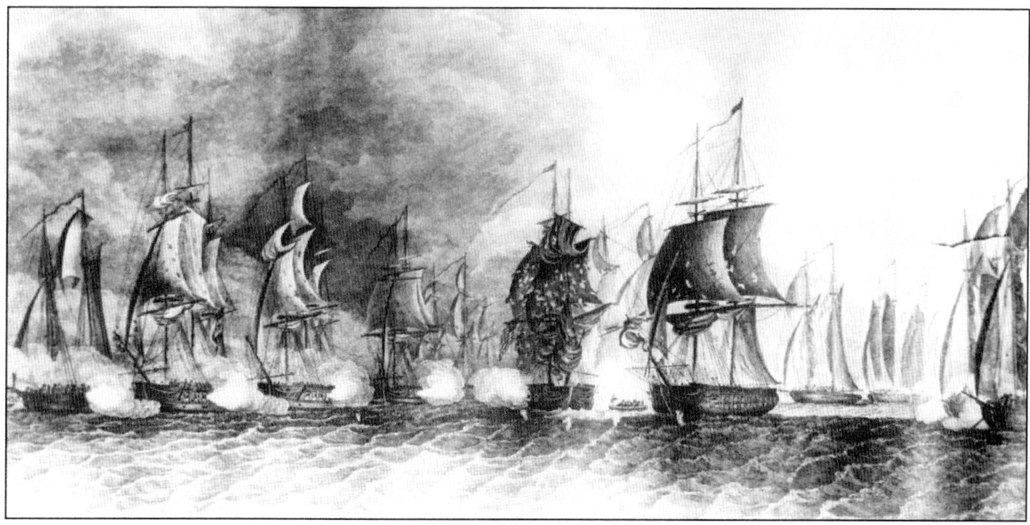

The Battle of Lake Erie was fought on September 10, 1813, during the War of 1812. Dr. Cyrenius Chapin was captured by the British and held in Montreal as a prisoner of war until his release in 1814. He returned to Buffalo to pursue his medical career. (Courtesy of the Buffalo History Museum, General Photograph Collection, Military–War of 1812.)

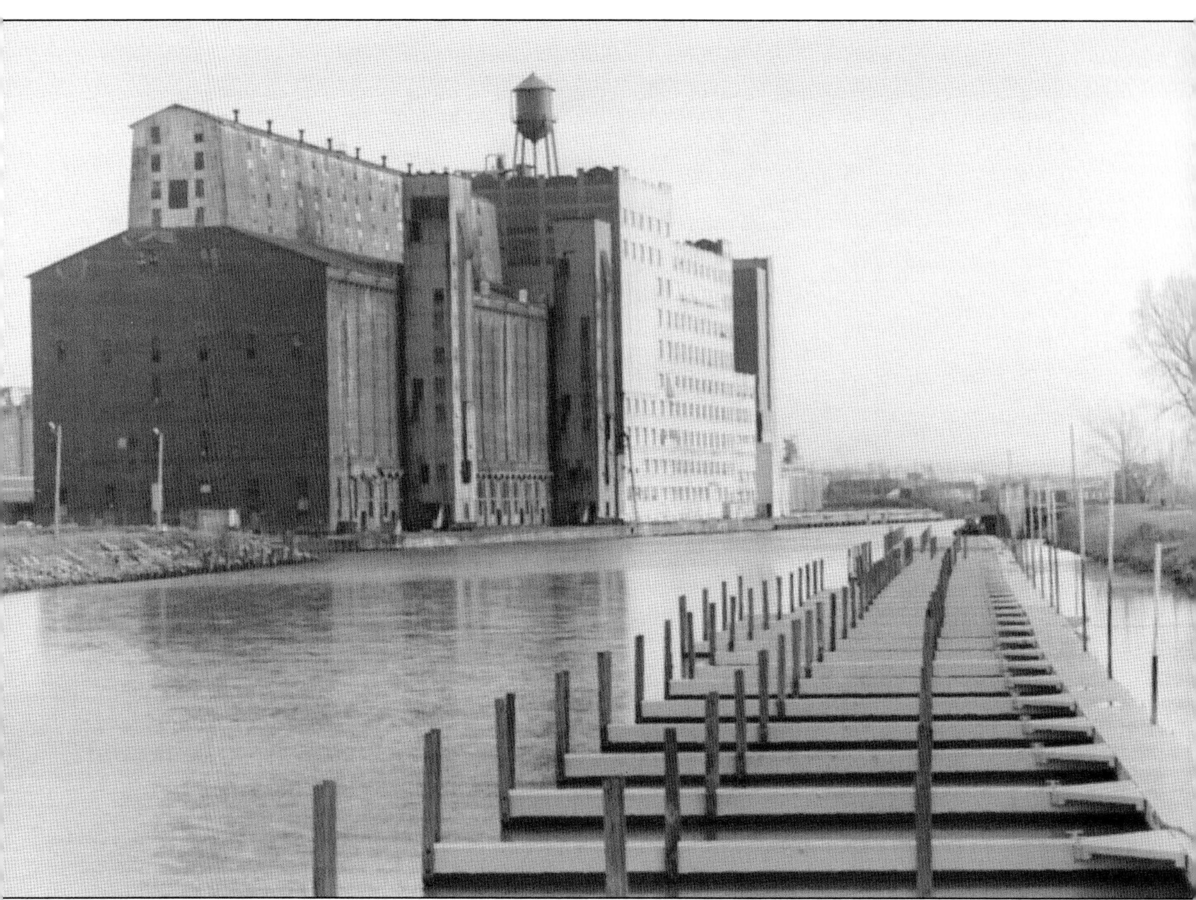

Construction of the Erie Canal began on July 4, 1817. It was built to create a navigable water route from New York City and the Atlantic Ocean to the Great Lakes, from the Hudson River to Lake Erie at Buffalo. The economic transformation provided by the canal contributed to medical innovation in the region. (Courtesy of University Archives, University at Buffalo.)

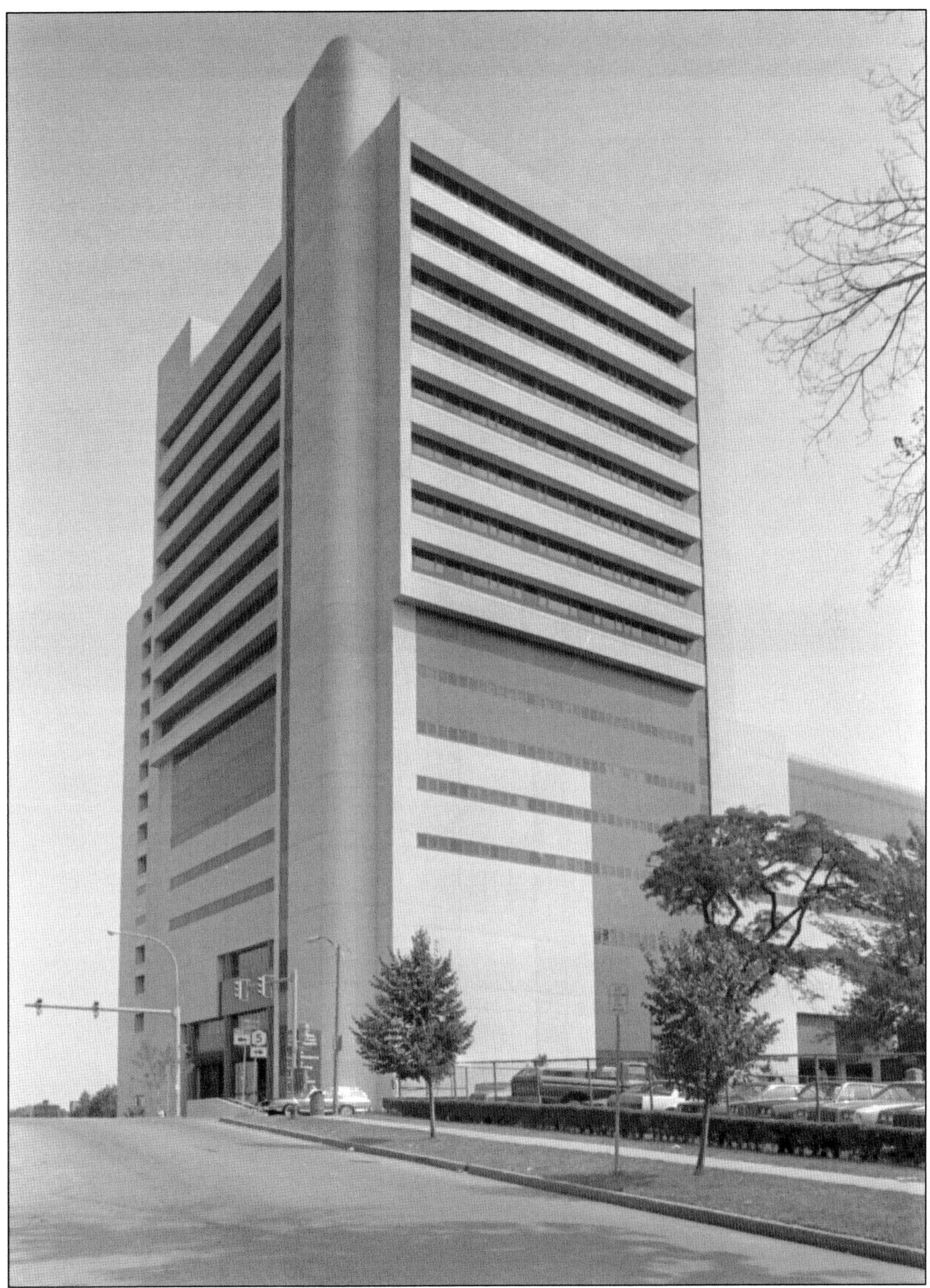

Buffalo General Hospital was established as a general public hospital in October 1846. Dr. Charles H. Wilcox, Medical Society of Erie County president in 1850, was a founding member of Buffalo General and the first medical officer from Buffalo to be commissioned during the Civil War. Dr. Wilcox died in 1862. (Courtesy of University Archives, University at Buffalo.)

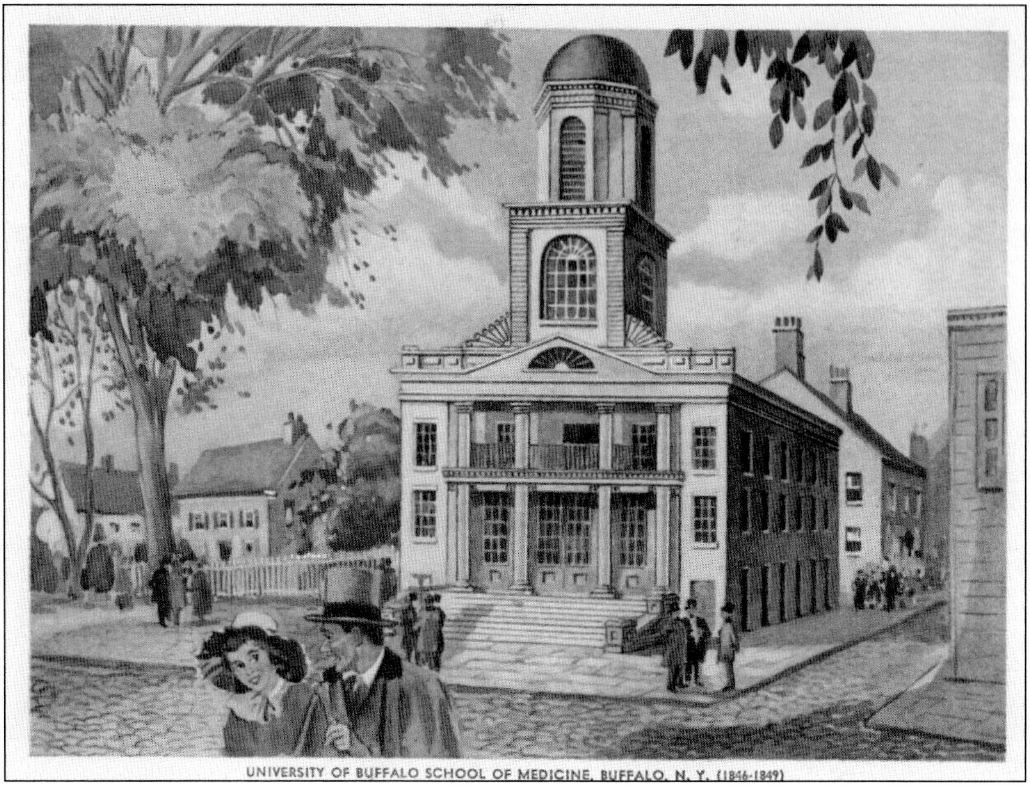

UNIVERSITY OF BUFFALO SCHOOL OF MEDICINE, BUFFALO, N. Y. (1846-1849)

This illustration depicts the University of Buffalo School of Medicine sometime between 1846 and 1849, when it was on Seneca and Washington Streets. This was the first site of the medical school founded by past Medical Society presidents Dr. Austin Flint (1858), Dr. James P. White (1855), and Dr. Frank Hamilton (1857). (Courtesy of University Archives, University at Buffalo.)

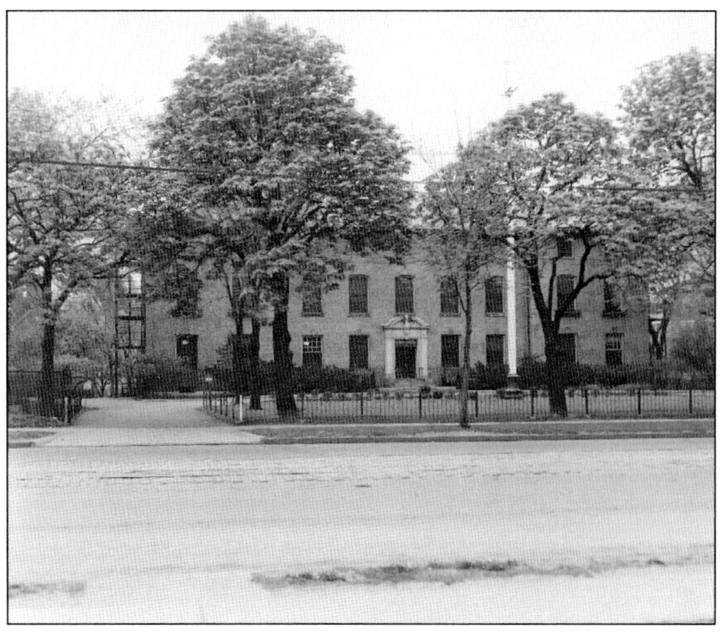

Pictured here is the Main Street campus of the University at Buffalo School of Medicine. Several past Medical Society presidents—Dr. James P. White (1855), Dr. Frank Hamilton (1857), and Dr. Austin Flint (1858)—were among the founders of the medical school. Sixty-six students registered for the first course of lectures, which began on February 24, 1847. (Courtesy of University Archives, University at Buffalo.)

Two

The Start of a Journey

As Erie County was experiencing a boom of growth and development, a new state law gave medical societies the legal authority to judge the fitness of physicians engaging in medical practice as well as the ability to set clinical, educational, and ethical standards of medical practice. The law set in motion the growth of medical societies as stewards of medical practices within their regions. The Medical Society of the County of Erie was founded in September 1821 as a means of fulfilling the legal requirement but also as a foundation for excellence in medical care, education, and innovation.

Erie County was the proud birthplace of many medical innovations, including the first implantable pacemaker, an infant screening test for phenylketonuria, an intrauterine birth control device, a drug designed to battle relapsing multiple sclerosis, and an artificial surfactant designed to save millions of infants from respiratory distress syndrome.

In addition to these many medical innovations, Erie County was the home of groundbreaking scientists who changed the face of medicine. Nobel Prize winners earning recognition for the discovery of the Cori cycle of metabolism and the transmission of chemical signals across nerve cell junctions called Buffalo home.

The Erie Canal was utilized as a mode of transportation from New York City to Buffalo, but for many residents, the railway was a superior means of travel. The Buffalo Railroad was chartered in 1833 and opened in 1834, operating a horse-driven line from downtown Buffalo to Black Rock. The Buffalo & Niagara Falls Railroad incorporated in 1834 to extend the railway north and northwest to Niagara Falls, and construction on the new railway began in August 1836. It extended the existing railway and also replaced the lower-quality rails of the horse-drawn lines.

The Erie Street Terminal was constructed in 1852 in the heart of downtown Buffalo. The New York Central Railroad formed in 1853 and leased the Buffalo & Niagara Falls Railroad, connecting them to New York City lines.

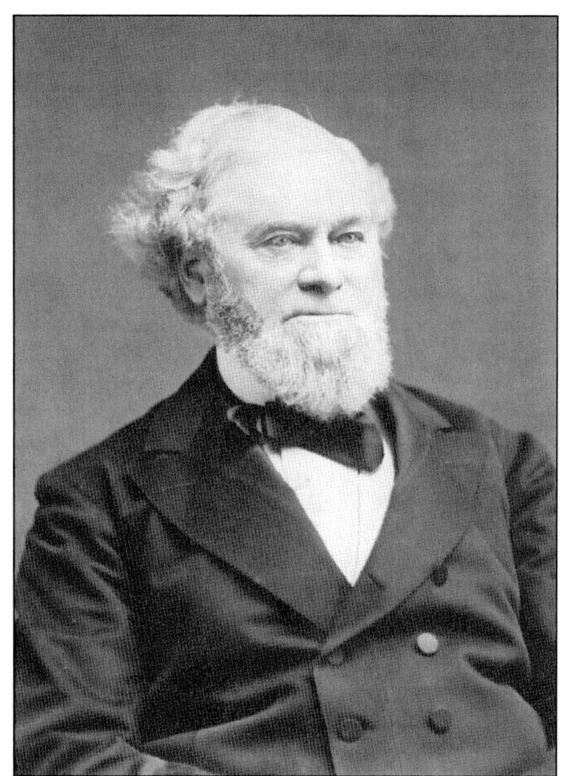

James Platt White, MD, the most noted obstetrician and gynecologist of his time, was the president of the Medical Society of Erie County in 1855 and held the same office in 1870. Dr. White, along with Dr. Austin Flint, was instrumental in founding the School of Medicine at the University of Buffalo and Buffalo Hospital of the Sisters of Charity. Dr. White was the inventor of obstetrical forceps and was among the first to use clinic instruction of medical students in the delivery of children. (Courtesy of the Buffalo History Museum, General Photograph Collection, Persons–W.)

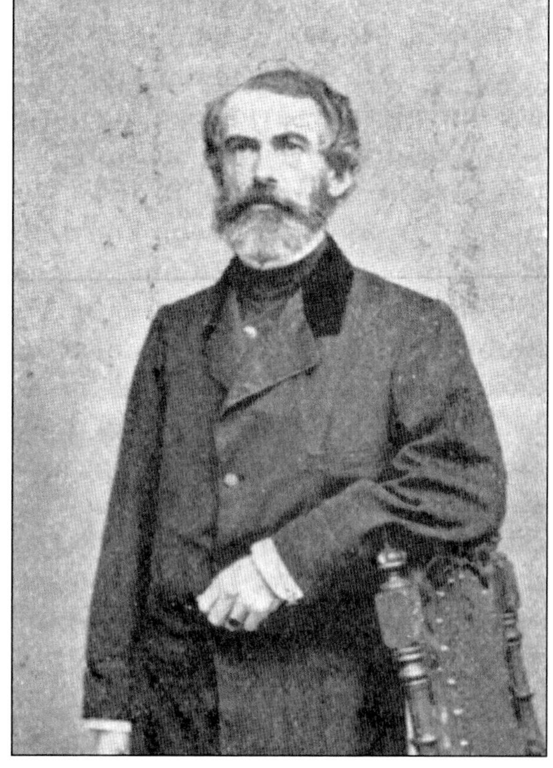

Frank Hamilton, MD, Medical Society of Erie County president in 1857, was one of the original faculty members at the University of Buffalo School of Medicine. Dr. Hamilton was the first person in western New York to perform plastic surgery, executing the first skin graft by transporting a piece of skin from a patient's left leg to an ulcer on his right leg. (Courtesy of the Buffalo History Museum, General Photograph Collection, Persons–H.)

Austin Flint, MD, arrived in Buffalo in 1836 and discovered the existence of typhoid fever in the county at North Boston. Dr. Flint was president of the Medical Society of Erie County in 1858 and practiced medicine in Buffalo until 1861. His numerous accomplishments include the founding of six medical schools, a medical journal, and a scientific society. (Courtesy of University Archives, University at Buffalo.)

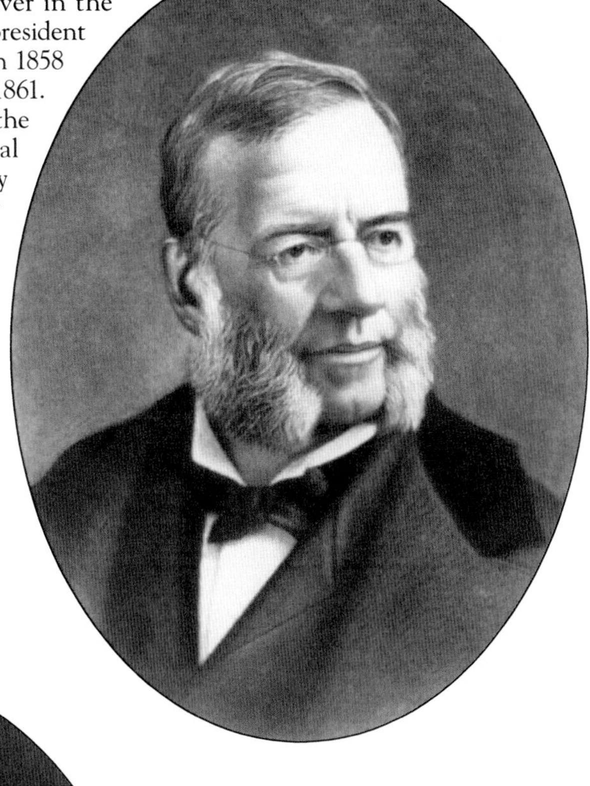

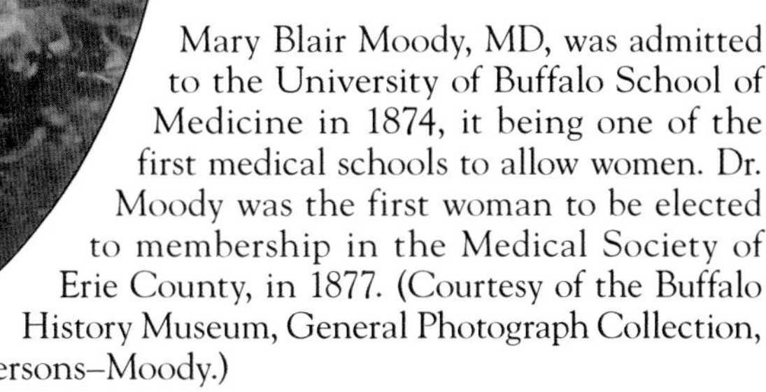

Mary Blair Moody, MD, was admitted to the University of Buffalo School of Medicine in 1874, it being one of the first medical schools to allow women. Dr. Moody was the first woman to be elected to membership in the Medical Society of Erie County, in 1877. (Courtesy of the Buffalo History Museum, General Photograph Collection, Persons–Moody.)

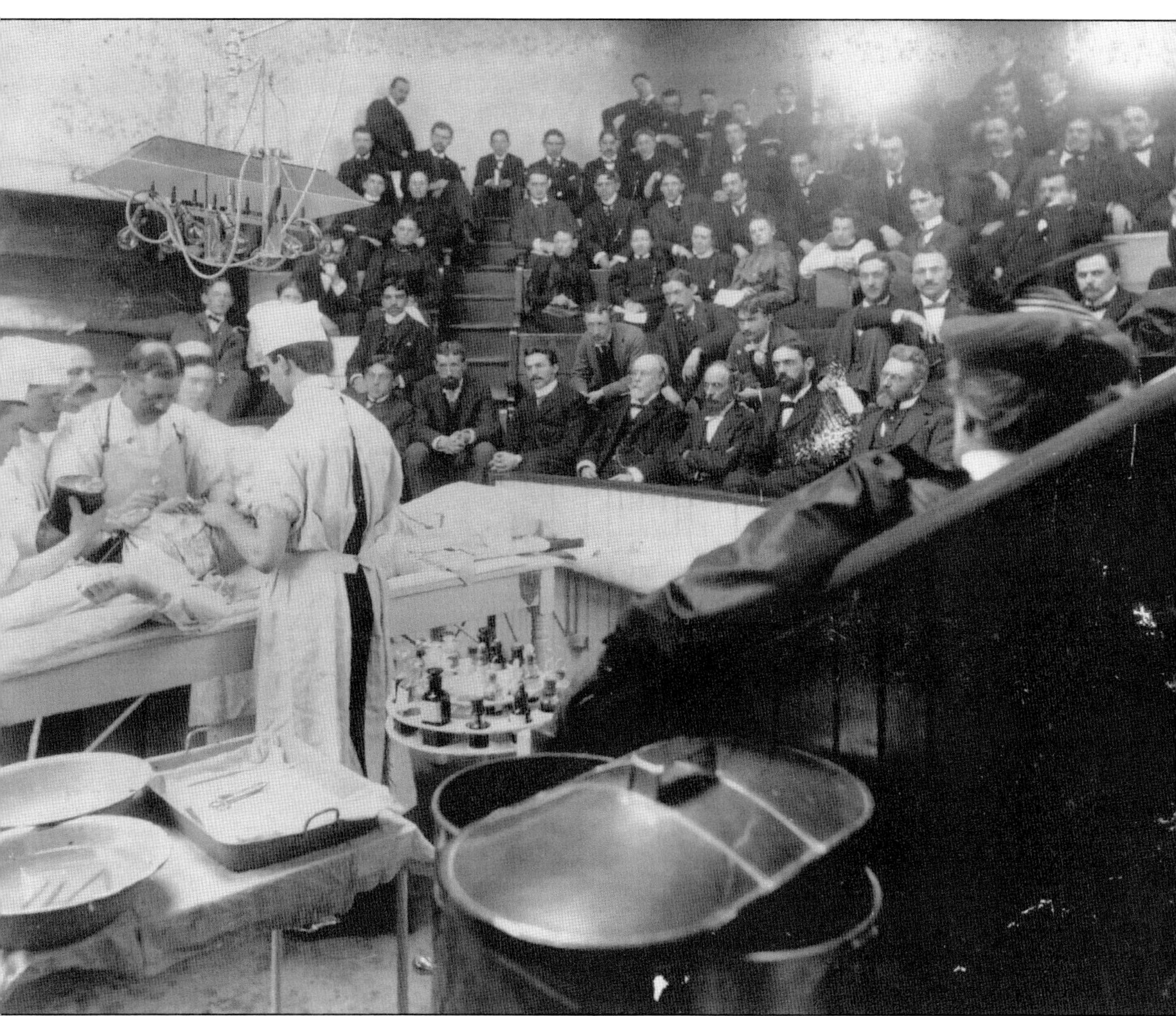

Pictured here is Dr. Roswell Park, professor of surgery at the University of Buffalo School of Medicine, in 1883. In 1891, Dr. Park came under heavy pressure to return to Chicago when he was asked to assume the chair of surgery at Rush Medical College, one of the most prestigious seats in the country. In a letter to the dean of Rush Medical College, Dr. Park explained that he had decided to remain in Buffalo due to his loyalty to the citizens and the profession of medicine in Buffalo. (Courtesy of University Archives, University at Buffalo.)

Three

Innovation, the Pandemic, and the Presidency

Hydroelectric power harnessed from the mighty Niagara Falls made Buffalo one of the first American cities to have electric lighting, resulting in Buffalo earning the nickname "City of Light." The power and beauty of electric lights were no better showcased than at the Pan-American Exposition in 1901. A surplus of this low-cost hydroelectric power propelled Buffalo to become a giant in the field of manufacturing.

The Pan-American Exposition was a world's fair that ran from May 1 through November 2, 1901. The fair stretched over 350 acres on the edge of Delaware Park. Buffalo was in competition with Niagara Falls over the honor to host the anticipated event. One reason for Buffalo's victory was its larger population; with over 350,000 people, it was the eighth-largest city in the United States at the time. A second reason was that Buffalo had better railroad connections, making access to the fair as easy as possible for many Americans.

The Pan-American Exposition is considered by many to be a high point for Buffalo, but unfortunately, it is more often remembered as the site where President McKinley was assassinated. While visiting the Temple of Music on September 6, 1901, the president was shot by anarchist Leon Czolgosz. McKinley died eight days later from gangrene caused by the bullet wounds. Many believed that Roswell Park, Buffalo's preeminent surgeon at the turn of the century, might have saved the president. But Park, who was in surgery in Niagara Falls when the shooting occurred, arrived too late to participate in the operation.

After the death of President McKinley, Vice Pres. Theodore Roosevelt took the oath of office at Buffalo's Wilcox Mansion.

Buffalo also has a connection to Millard Fillmore, the 13th president of the United States. Fillmore was a native of East Aurora and served as the first chancellor of the University of Buffalo. Grover Cleveland, the 22nd and 24th president, started his political career in Buffalo. Cleveland served both as Erie County sheriff and mayor of Buffalo prior to his rise into national politics.

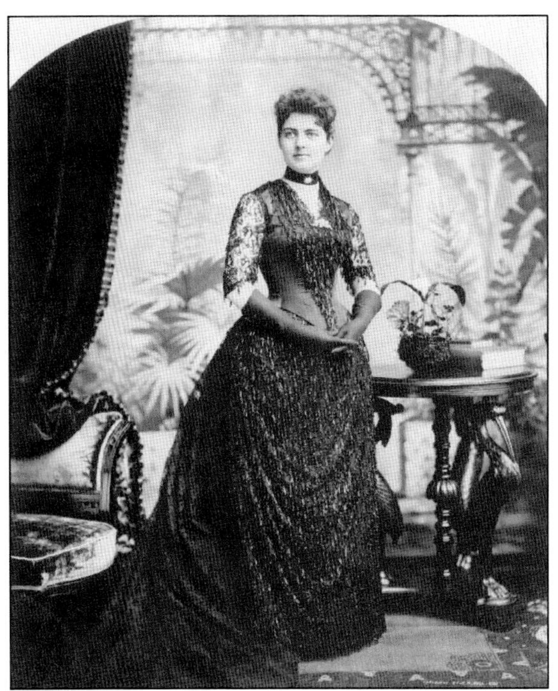

Frances Folsom, born in Buffalo, was the youngest first lady of the United States at age 21, from 1886 to 1889 and again from 1893 to 1897, and remains so to this day. Her husband, Grover Cleveland, was the mayor of Buffalo in 1882. Their baby Ruth died of diphtheria in 1904. At that time, Buffalo health commissioner Earnest Wende emerged as a public health leader and founded Earnest Wende Hospital, dedicated to the treatment of infectious diseases such as diphtheria. (Courtesy of the Buffalo History Museum, General Photograph Collection, Grover Cleveland photographic collection, Box 1, Folder 35.)

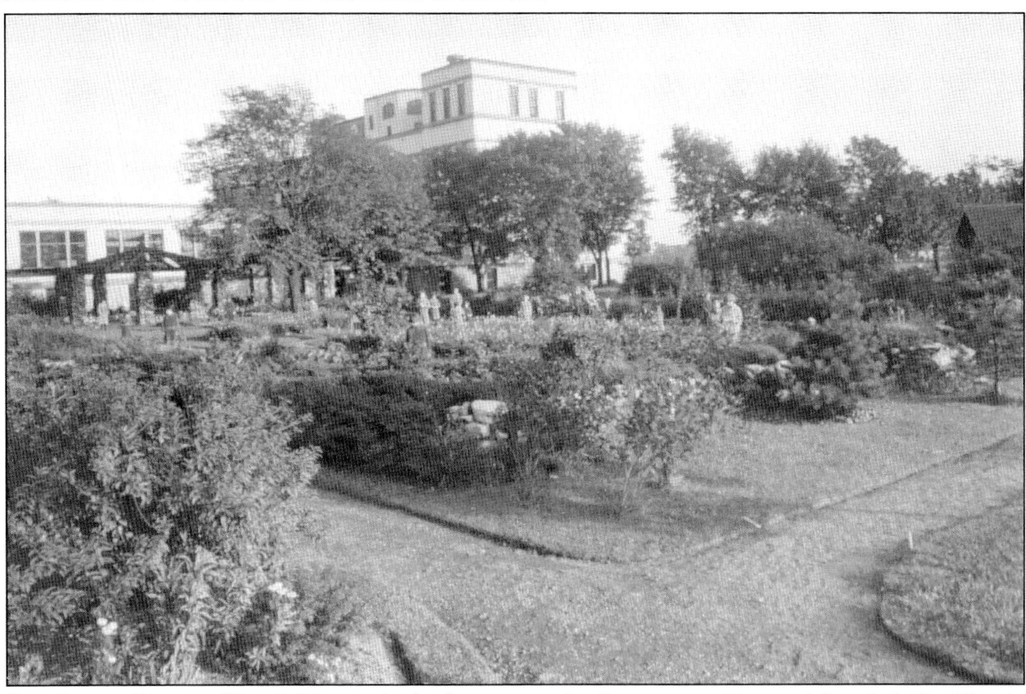

Seen here is Earnest Wende Hospital, also known as the Contagious Disease Hospital. Dr. Wende was president of the Medical Society of Erie County in 1903 and Buffalo city health commissioner from 1892 to 1901 and 1907 to 1910. During his tenure, the death rate in Buffalo was the lowest of any city of its size in the world. Dr. Wende graduated from the University of Buffalo in 1878 and was credited with determining the source of the typhoid fever epidemic. (Courtesy of University Archives, University at Buffalo.)

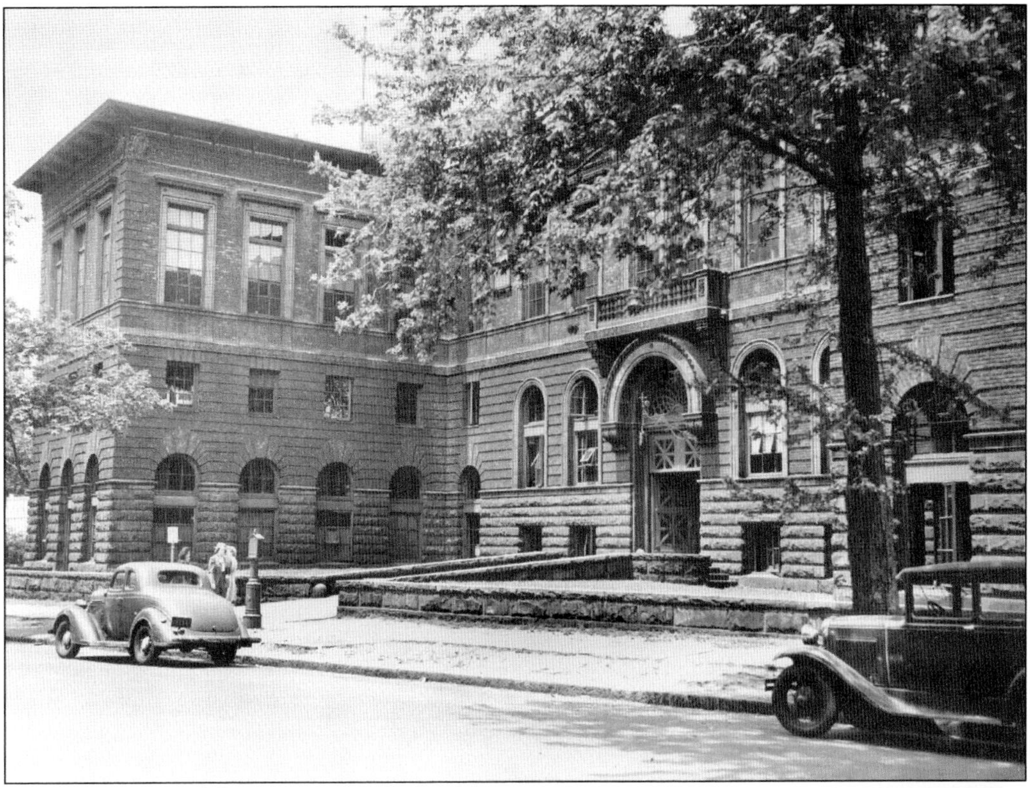

The third home of the University of Buffalo School of Medicine (1893–1954) was at 24 High Street. When the main university campus was moved to Main Street in the 1920s, the School of Medicine remained downtown near Buffalo General Hospital. (Courtesy of University Archives, University at Buffalo.)

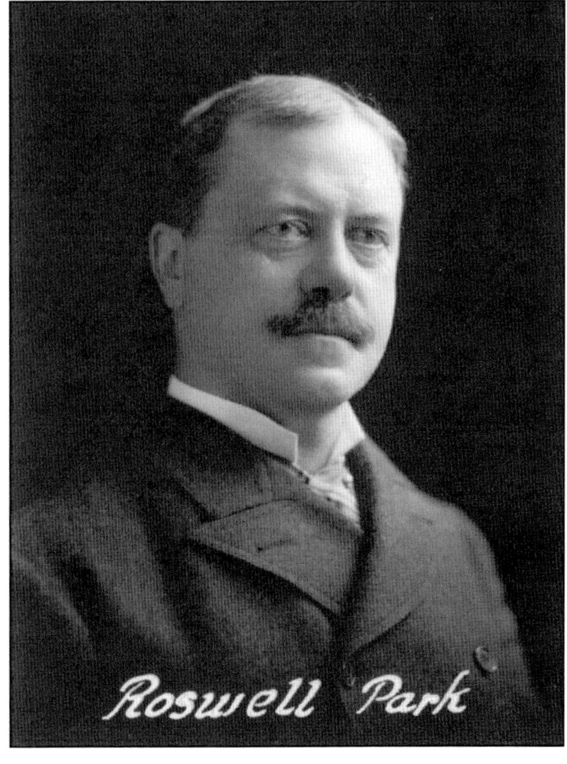

One of the most prominent American surgeons is Dr. Roswell Park, who came to Buffalo in 1883 to be a surgery professor at the University of Buffalo. Shortly after his arrival, Dr. Park became chief of surgery at Buffalo General Hospital. He was best known for starting the New York State Pathological Laboratory in 1898, which was later expanded into the Gratwick Research Laboratory and is now known as the Roswell Park Comprehensive Cancer Center. (Courtesy of the Buffalo History Museum, General Photograph Collection, Persons–P.)

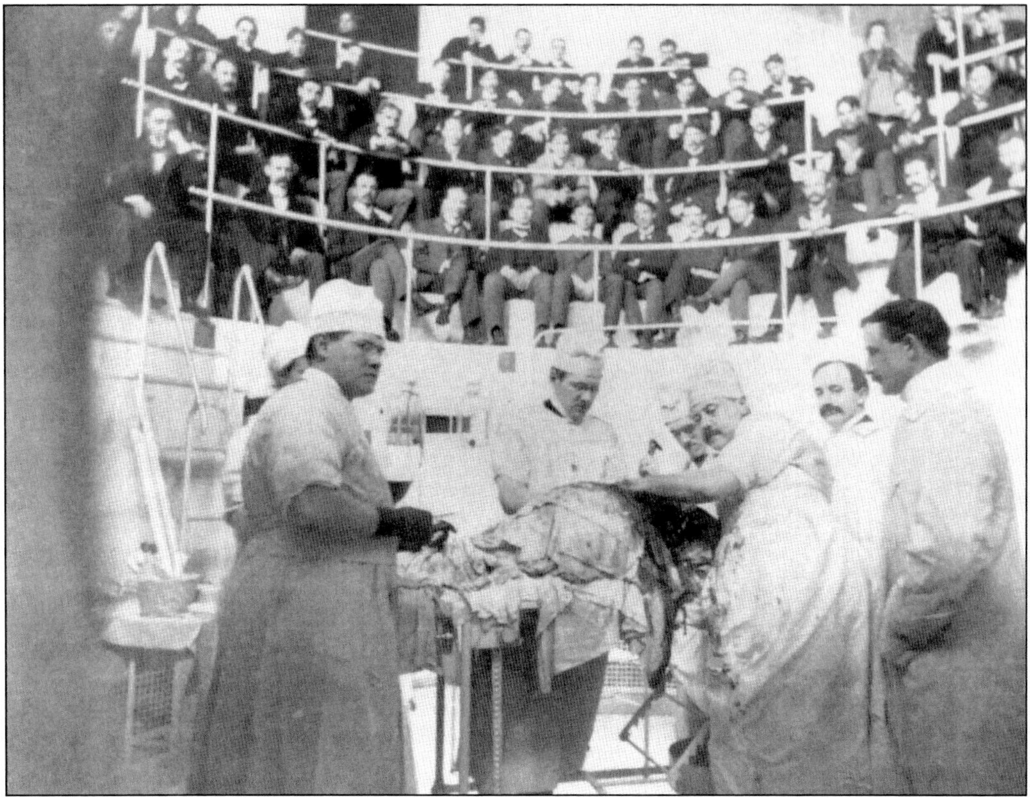

Roswell Park performs surgery before medical students. Dr. Park served as professor of surgery at the University of Buffalo School of Medicine. His greatest ambition was to discover the cause of cancer, and he received grant money in 1898 from the state legislature to establish the New York State Pathological Laboratory, the world's first laboratory devoted to cancer research. It is known today as the Roswell Park Comprehensive Care Center. (Courtesy of University Archives, University at Buffalo.)

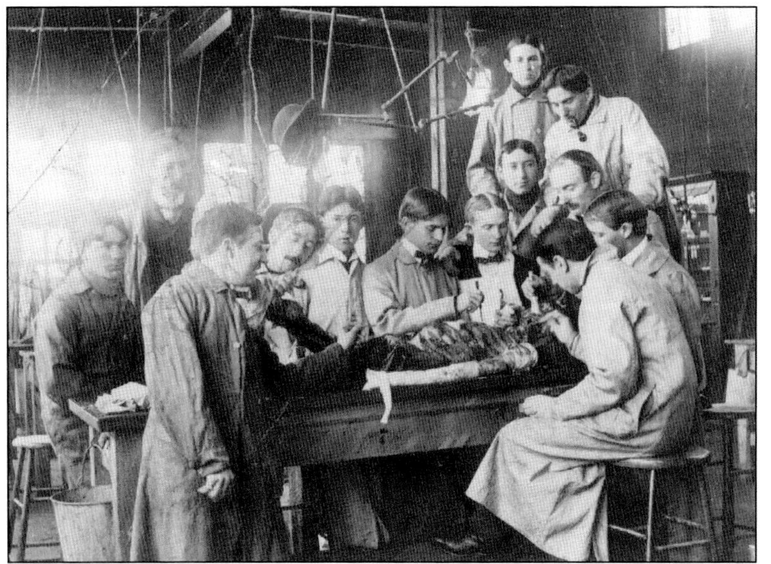

Buffalo medical students are gathered around a body in 1900. At this time, Buffalo was the eighth-largest city in the nation and just three years earlier had been selected to host the prestigious Pan-American Exposition in 1897, a showcase for new technology. (Courtesy of University Archives, University at Buffalo.)

Dr. Earnest Wende, credited with determining the source of the typhoid fever epidemic, also initiated several innovative ideas while he was health commissioner: contagious diseases were reported by phone at the city's expense, houses where people with contagious diseases lived were given medical and sanitary inspections, wells were systematically examined and closed if necessary, and the health office was open 24 hours to receive complaints, grant permits, and act in urgent cases.

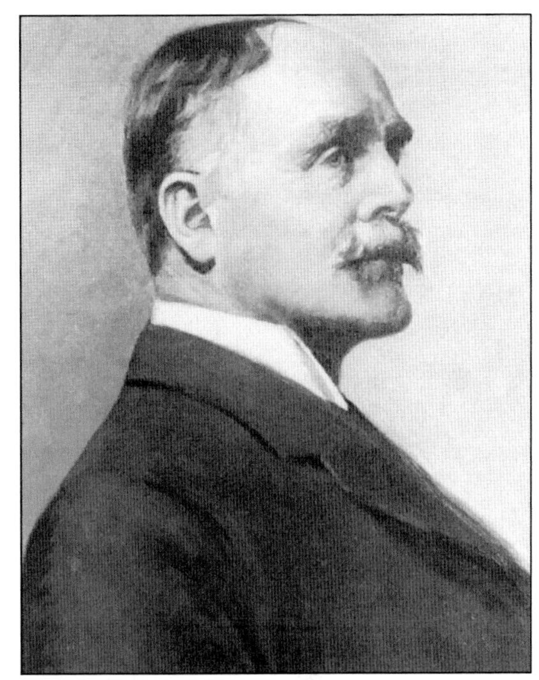

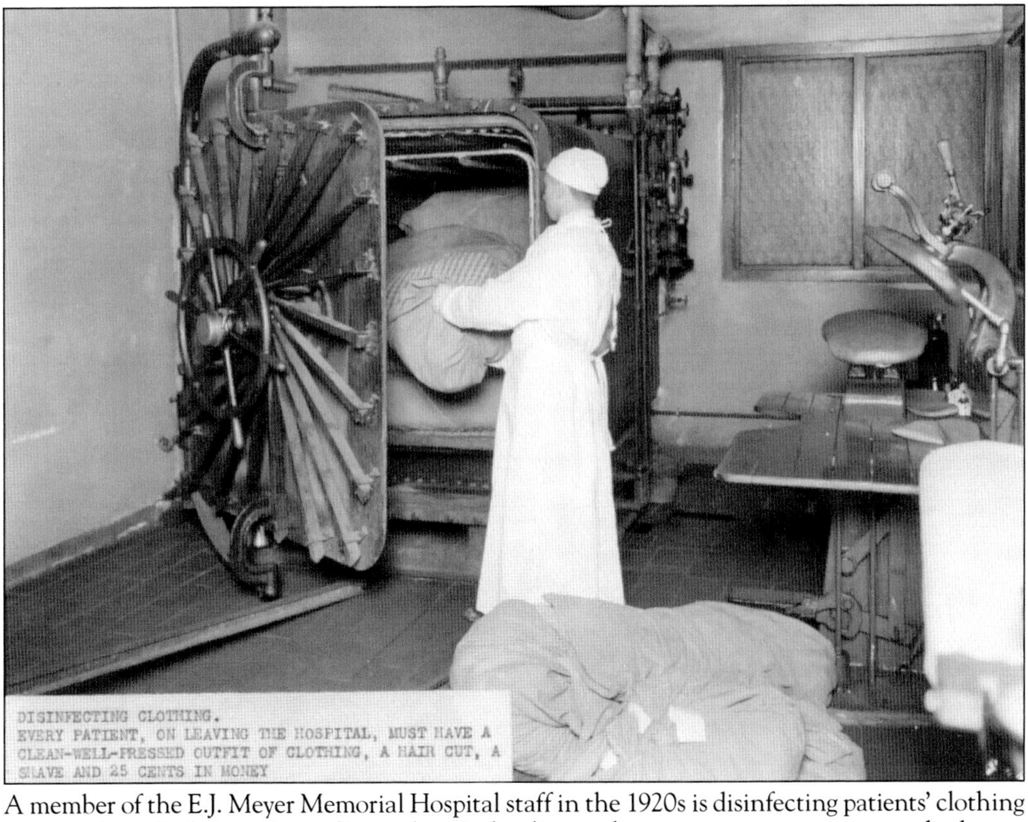

A member of the E.J. Meyer Memorial Hospital staff in the 1920s is disinfecting patients' clothing prior to their discharge. According to hospital policy at the time, every patient, upon discharge, was provided a clean, well-pressed outfit of clothing, a haircut, a shave, and 25¢.

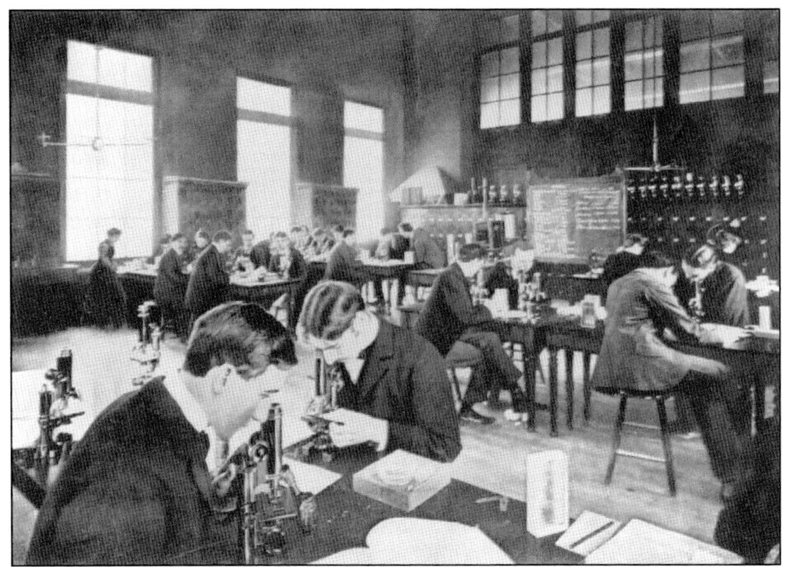

The High Street location of the medical laboratory at the University of Buffalo School of Medicine is seen here. After four decades at Main and Virginia Streets, a block on High Street was purchased for the new School of Medicine location. (Courtesy of University Archives, University at Buffalo.)

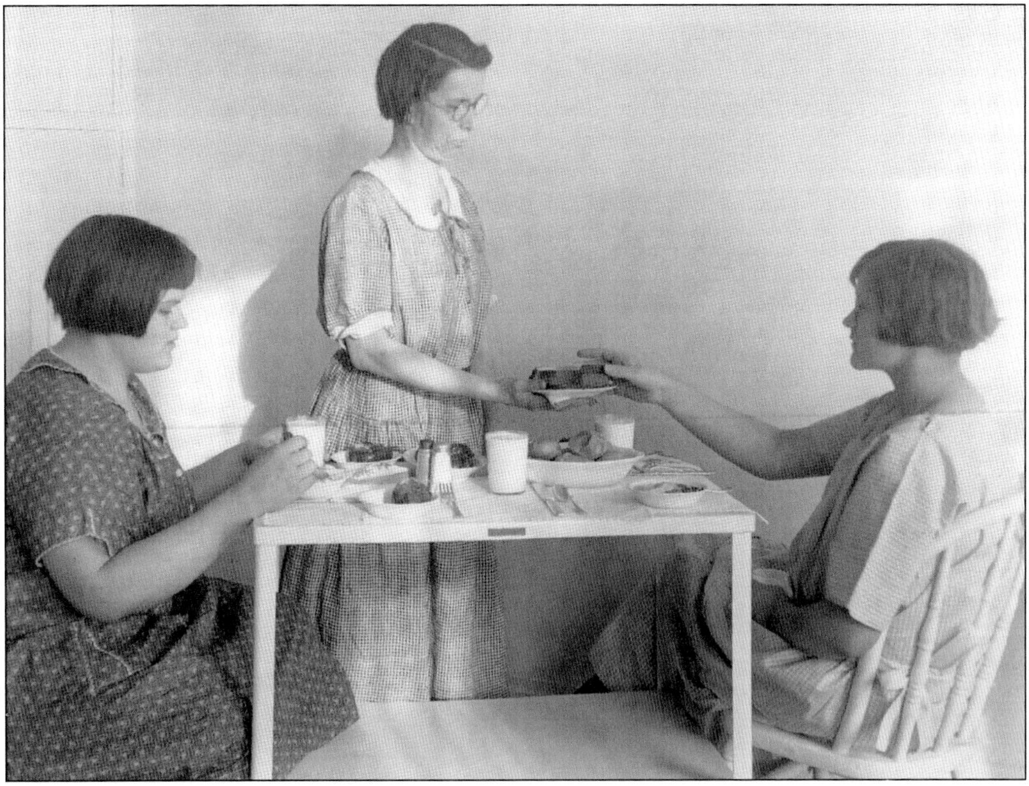

Found in the Medical Society of Erie County archives was this picture labeled "Unwed Mothers at Breakfast," referencing women during their stay at the Mother Theresa Home: Haven for Single Mothers. (Courtesy of the Buffalo History Museum, General Photograph Collection, Social Services–Maternity Homes.)

This December 1927 Medical Society of Erie County *Bulletin* advertisement expresses appreciation for medical professionals for preventing the "great white plague" and issues a call for society members to appear for professional photographs for the fourth volume of the Portrait Library of the Medical Society of Erie County.

WE take this opportunity to thank members of the medical profession who have contributed so liberally to the distribution of

Tuberculosis Christmas Seals

and have commended our methods of preventing the spread of the great white plague.

Buffalo Tuberculosis Association

175 Swan Street Buffalo, N. Y.

1927

Christmas Greetings and Good Health

ATTENTION OF NEW MEMBERS!

We are completing the fourth volume of the Portrait Library of the Medical Society of the County of Erie.

Appointments for sittings should be made not later than January 1, 1928.

JUANITA BALL STUDIO

Official Photographer for Medical Society

640 MAIN ST. Telehone Tupper 0284 BUFFALO

The Approaching Danger Months

Chart shows the Annual Death-rate per 100,000 of Buffalo Population over a period of Three Years.

Month	Death-rate
July	45
Aug.	49
Sept.	43
Oct.	79
Nov.	135
Dec.	134
Jan.	131
Feb.	143
Mar.	213
Apr.	210
May	147

Maximum Protection to Patients is Provided in Our HEATED Invalid Coaches, Extra All-wool Blankets, Hot-water Bottles and doors weather-stripped against drafts.

MASON-HEYL Inc. **Crescent 7210**

OPERATING AMBULANCE SERVICE FOR:

DEACONESS, LAFAYETTE GENERAL, LADY OF VICTORY, U. S. MARINE HOSPITALS.

Parkside Sanitarium and Hospital 1392 AMHERST ST. BUFFALO, N. Y.

A Homelike Institution for the Care and Treatment of

NERVOUS DISEASES INVALIDISM AGED PEOPLE

We accept patients who do not do well at home. They are cared for under the direction of the Family Physician.

OPENED 1902 Sidney A. Dunham, M. D., Superintendent.

PLEASE NOTE: *Advertisers are demonstrating a splendid spirit of co-operation to help defray the cost of publishing your* BULLETIN. *Patronize the friends of organized medicine and let them know they are getting direct results.*

December, 1927 *BULLETIN* 9

PAY YOUR STATE REGISTRATION FEE BEFORE DECEMBER 31!

Annual registration forms, sent to licensed physicians last October by the State Department of Education, should be returned to Albany not later than December 31, accompanied with the two dollar fee, in order to be exempt from payment of a further fee of one dollar for each thirty days or part thereof that the physician is in default. Compliance with this requirement insures the insertion of the doctor's name and address in the 1928 list of medical practitioners entitled to engage in practice in New York State. Physicians who were registered last year do not require the certification of a notary for re-registration. If you have not received or have mislaid your blank, apply at once to the Secretary of the State Board of Medical Examiners, Education Building, Albany, N. Y.

REYNOLDS, LABORATORY FAKER, AGAIN JAILED

The Journal of the American Medical Association for November 19th, quoting Ohio newspapers, reports that Horace D. Reynolds was being held in Cleveland without bond when two victims died and four others became seriously ill following the administration of Reynolds' so-called serum.

Reynolds and his son-in-law, George H. Harris, are not strangers to the police authorities of Buffalo. For several months the pair operated the "Buffalo Research Laboratory" in the Walbridge Building and announced a cure for a variety of physical disorders. The extraordinary statements made in their newspaper advertisements brought them in conflict with the Buffalo Better Business Bureau. It was learned that Old Doc Reynolds had been arrested in various cities, and had been driven out of Chicago, in 1926, following exposure by the Chicago Tribune. Suave yet defiant, Reynolds invited the closest scrutiny of his methods of treatment in Buffalo. The offer was accepted and the office files of the concern were examined by representatives of the Better Business Bureau. The names of a dozen or more alleged patients, mostly women, were obtained. A check-up disclosed that these persons were employed by Reynolds to boost his business among their neighbors and bring in new patients.

The advertising bait of the "Buffalo Research Laboratory" was the phrase "Blood or Urinalysis $1.00." It brought a stream of credulous persons to the office, where the doctor in charge promptly separated the victims from sums ranging from $5.00 to $100.00. Circulars exposing the fraud partly stopped the rush. Finally, evidence was obtained that prompted Reynolds to leave town, and the place was permanently closed February 12, 1927, after Harris had been arrested and fined on a minor charge.

The article in the Journal of the A. M. A. observes that advertising quacks "can be driven out of a city either by a newspaper or a Better Business Bureau that will investigate the methods and give the public the facts." The latter method has been employed in Buffalo repeatedly with marked success.

C. W. BETHUNE, M. D.

UROLOGICAL STAFF MEETINGS AT BUFFALO CITY HOSPITAL

Staff meetings in Urology will be held the second Tuesday of each month from December to April, inclusive, at the Buffalo City Hospital, to which all the physicians in Erie County, who may be interested, are cordially invited. The chief urologist is Dr. F. J. Parmenter; associates are: Drs. Oberkircher, Watson, Slotkin, Martin, Leutenegger and Kutzman.

The first of this series of urological staff meetings was held Tuesday,

A December 1927 *Bulletin* announcement reads that Horace Reynolds and his son-in-law George Harris, who operated the Buffalo Research Laboratory, were held in Cleveland, Ohio, "without bond when two victims died and four others became seriously ill following the administration of Reynolds' so-called serum."

4 BULLETIN June, 1928

BUFFALO DOCTORS HONORED

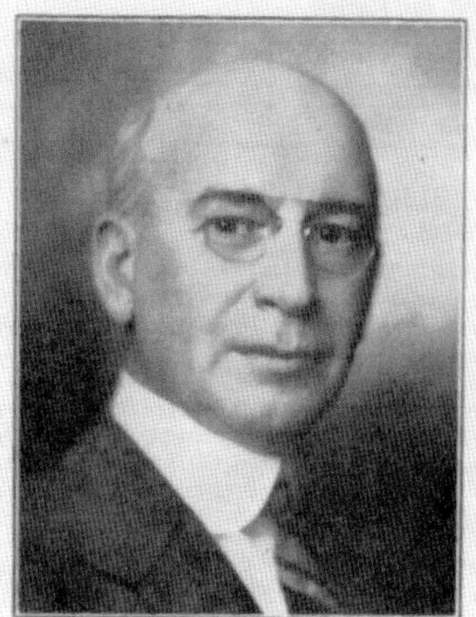

DR. HARRY R. TRICK
President of the Medical Society of the State of New York. Installed at Annual Meeting in Albany, May 21, 1928.

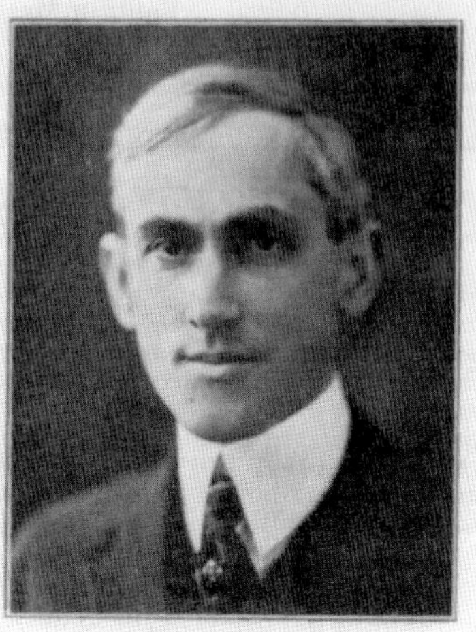

DR. EDWARD WILLIAM KOCH
Chosen Acting Dean of the School of Medicine of the University of Buffalo.

At left is Dr. Harry Trick, Buffalo physician and member of the Medical Society of Erie County. Dr. Trick served as president of the Medical Society of the State of New York in 1928. Also pictured is Dr. Edward William Koch, who served as acting dean of the University of Buffalo School of Medicine. (Courtesy of University Archives, University at Buffalo.)

June, 1928 BULLETIN 5

HARRY RADLEY TRICK, M. D., F. A. C. S.

Dr. Harry R. Trick was installed President of the Medical Society of the State of New York at the one hundred and twenty-second annual meeting, held at Albany, May 21 to 24, and attended by about one thousand physicians.

Dr. Trick was graduated from the School of Medicine of the University of Buffalo, in 1901, and for many years has been prominently identified with activities of organized medicine. He is a former President of the Buffalo Academy of Medicine, and for six years was President of the Eighth District Branch of the State Medical Society. In 1926 he was elevated to the position of Vice-Speaker of the House of Delegates of the State Medical Society, and in 1927 he was chosen President-elect. In his Presidential greetings Dr. Trick stated that the last five years have seen a great broadening of the field of the Society, especially in the assumption of leadership in all civic duties in which health is involved. He declared that the President must now deal with governmental officials and civic organizations as well as with physicians, and must make the discharge of his society duties the predominant object of his daily work.

Dr. Trick is a member of the Executive Committee of the School of Medicine of the University of Buffalo; Professor of Surgery at that institution, and a member of the surgical staffs of the Buffalo General Hospital, Buffalo City Hospital and Buffalo State Hospital.

EDWARD WILLIAM KOCH, A. M., M. D.

Dr. Edward W. Koch, who for the past ten years has been head of the Department of Pharmacology and Secretary of the School of Medicine of the University of Buffalo, has been chosen Acting Dean of the School of Medicine by the Council, to succeed the late Dr. C. Sumner Jones.

Dr. Koch received the degree of Master of Arts from Indiana University, and was graduated in medicine from Rush Medical College in 1911. For a number of years he was engaged in teaching in the School of Medicine of Indiana University, and subsequently was pharmacologist for Eli Lilly & Company.

The experience acquired by Dr. Koch as a member of the Executive Committee; the Board of Instruction, and Professor of Pharmacology of the School of Medicine of the University of Buffalo are among the qualifications that fit him for his new administrative duties.

WILLIAM F. JACOBS, M. D.

Dr. William F. Jacobs, a trustee of the Buffalo Academy of Medicine for the past three years, was elected President of that scientific body at the annual meeting held May 13th. He succeeds Dr. George J. Eckel.

Dr. Jacobs was graduated from the School of Medicine of the University of Buffalo in 1908. He served his interneship at the Buffalo General Hospital and soon thereafter began specialization in pathology, acquiring further knowledge at world-famous clinics in Europe. In 1921 Dr. Jacobs joined the staff of the Buffalo City Hospital to take charge of the pathological department. He is Professor of pathology at the School of Medicine of

The Medical Society of Erie County *Bulletin* in June 1928 highlighted the accomplishments of Erie County physician members Harry Trick, MD; Edward William Koch, MD; and William F. Jacobs, MD. Dr. Jacobs graduated from the University of Buffalo School of Medicine in 1908, joined the staff of Buffalo City Hospital in 1921 as the head of the pathology department, and was elected president of the scientific body of the Buffalo Academy of Medicine in May 1928.

Four

Women in the Society and the Society *Bulletin*

On August 18, 1920, the 19th Amendment to the US Constitution granted women in the United States the right to vote. Notably, women's rights were also beginning to take shape at the Medical Society of Erie County at that time.

Just eight years after the passing of the 19th Amendment, Dr. Louise Beamis and Dr. Mary Kazmierczak were elected the first female officers of the Medical Society. Dr. Beamis was installed as secretary, and Dr. Kazmierczak was selected as one of eight delegates from Erie County after a majority vote at the state medical society annual meeting.

During this time, the Medical Society *Bulletin* became an important source of information, from advertisements featuring the latest medical products and devices to notices on how to support the World War I effort by purchasing US savings bonds.

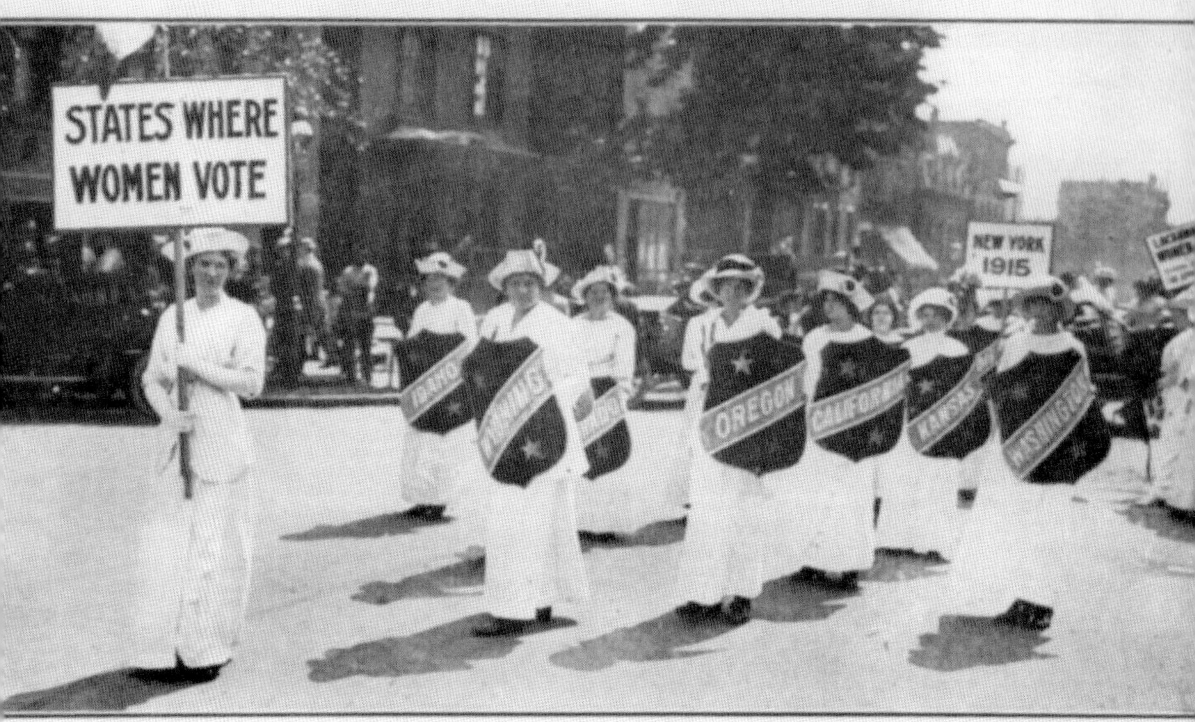

STATES WHERE WOMEN VOTE: A SECTION IN THE WOMAN SUFFRAGE PARADE

Just 10 years before Dr. Louise Beamis and Dr. Mary Kazmierczak were elected the first female officers of the Medical Society of Erie County in 1928, the women pictured here marched in the streets of New York City seeking the right to vote. (Courtesy of the Buffalo History Museum, General Photograph Collection, Political Movements.)

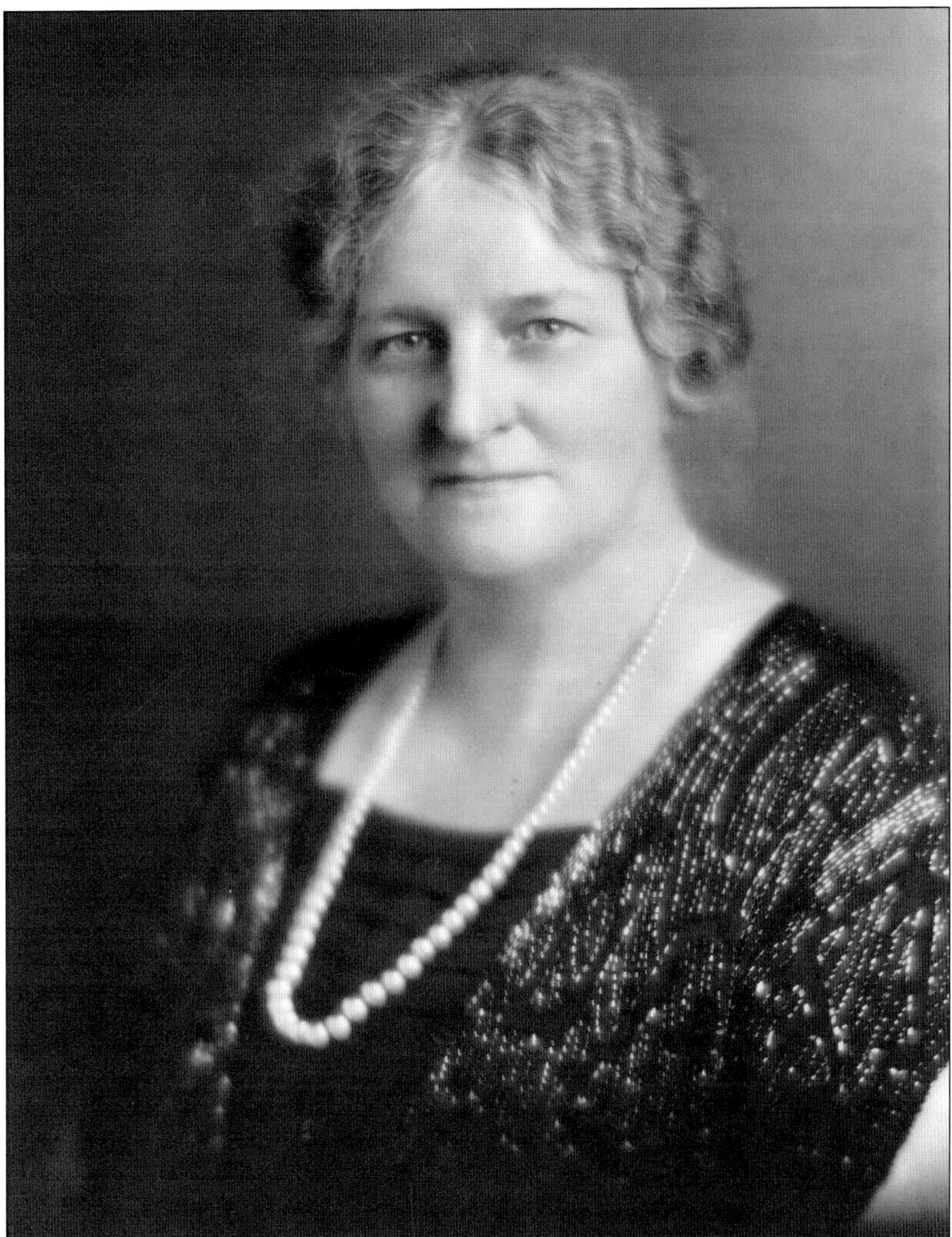

Dr. Louise Beamis was the first woman physician to be elected as an officer to the Medical Society of Erie County, on December 17, 1928; she held the position of secretary. This was a remarkable feat considering it came just eight years after the enactment of the 19th Amendment, which granted women in the United States the right to vote. (Photograph by Juanita Ball.)

February, 1929 5

DR. DE CEU HEADS MERCY HOSPITAL STAFF

Dr. Robert E. De Ceu, 40 Indian Church Road, was elected and installed President of the Mercy Hospital staff at its meeting February 5. Dr. De Ceu is a former President of the Medical Society of the County of Erie, and one of the most active workers in promoting the scientific and economic programs of the local bodies of the organized medical profession.

CLINICAL INFORMATION

Arrangements are under way by the Bulletin Publication Committee and the superintendents of the various hospitals in Buffalo, whereby physicians and surgeons visiting this city can be informed of the hour of holding clinics and the nature of the operations, by telephoning Jefferson 10,000. It is hoped this system may develop into a daily bulletin of opportunities for clinical study and add to Buffalo's fame as a medical and surgical center.

"DROPPED FOR NON-PAYMENT OF DUES!"

The treasurer of almost every medical organization with a large membership roll is obliged to note in his annual report the names of members dropped for non-payment of dues—a duty none too pleasant.

Requests for reinstatement are frequent, and in county medical societies the application usually involves a great deal of time and considerable correspondence, particularly if the applicant has been a non-member a year or more, before correct information regarding eligibility can be obtained for consideration by the society.

The Bulletin of the Cleveland Academy of Medicine, under the caption *"Locking the Barn,"* cites several excellent reasons for maint[illegible]ning membership unbroken at all times in a county medical society:

Membership in many national medical bodies, particularly t[illegible]er-ican Medical Association, is contingent on membership in the [illegible]ical society of the county where the physician resides.

Medical defense, provided by the State Medical Society, lapses immediately on failure to pay dues on time.

Opportunities to present scientific papers are scarce unless membership in the county medical society is maintained.

Many positions with insurance companies and industrial plants are open only to members of a county medical society.

Membership in a county medical society is evidence in itself of a desire on the part of the physician to affiliate himself with the most progressive elements in the profession.

Membership is an indication that the physician is contributing to the field of public relationship by being interested in an organization which is constantly at work to better the relationship between medicine, the public and the official branches of government.

Membership is an indication to those who seek information about him that he has the best interest of his profession at heart.

Membership indicates that the physician is in touch with the newest advances in medicine through attendance at meetings of his county medical or allied organizations.

Membership unbroken indicates that the physician is desirous of maintaining his standing locally.

A February 1929 *Bulletin* advertisement honors the former president of the Medical Society and founder of the Mercy Hospital staff, Dr. Robert De Ceu. Dr. De Ceu was a prominent advocate for organized medicine. Also in this issue was a section listing the value-add of membership to the Medical Society.

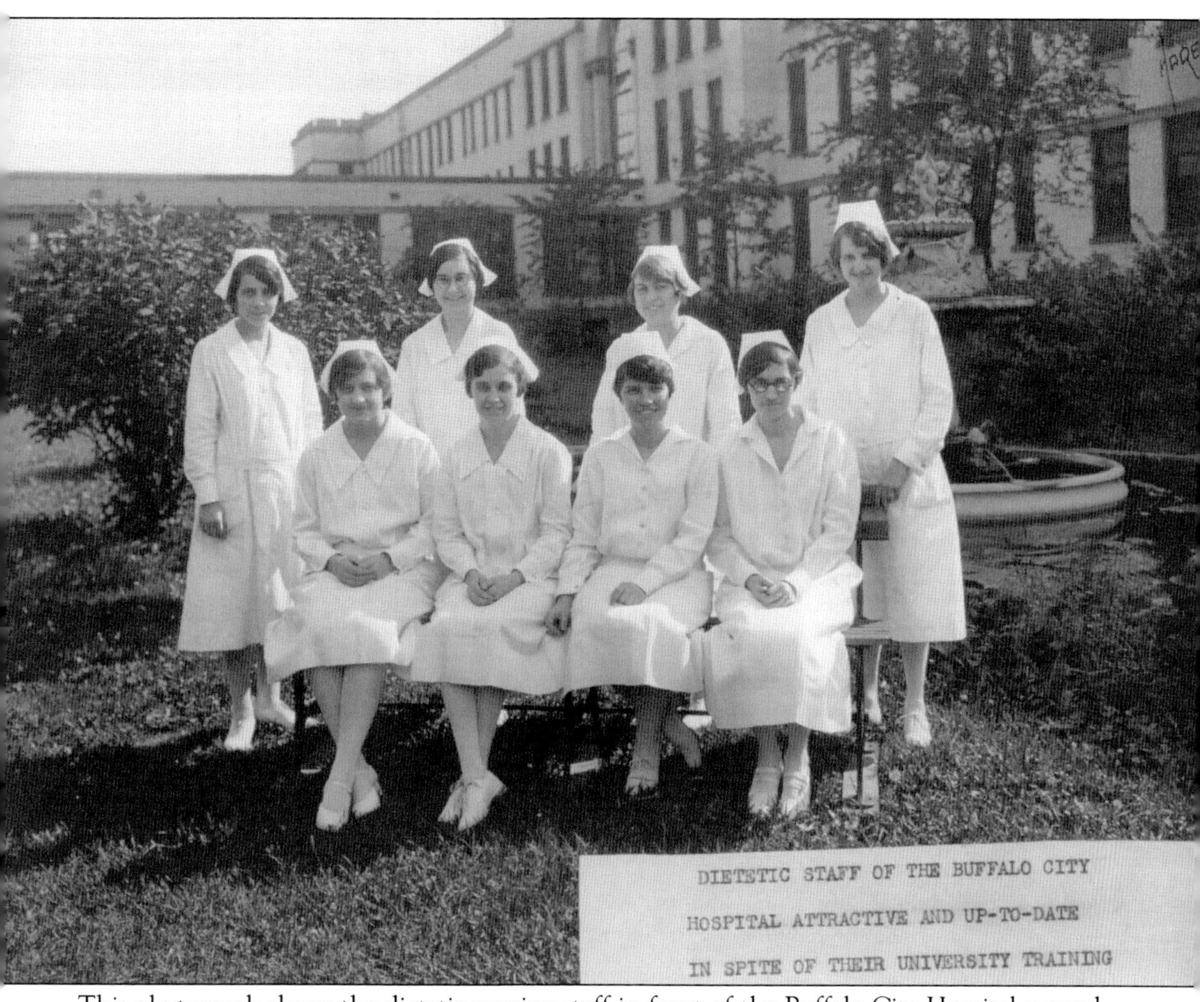

This photograph shows the dietetic nursing staff in front of the Buffalo City Hospital around 1929. The caption reads, "Dietetic staff of the Buffalo City Hospital attractive and up-to-date in spite of their university training."

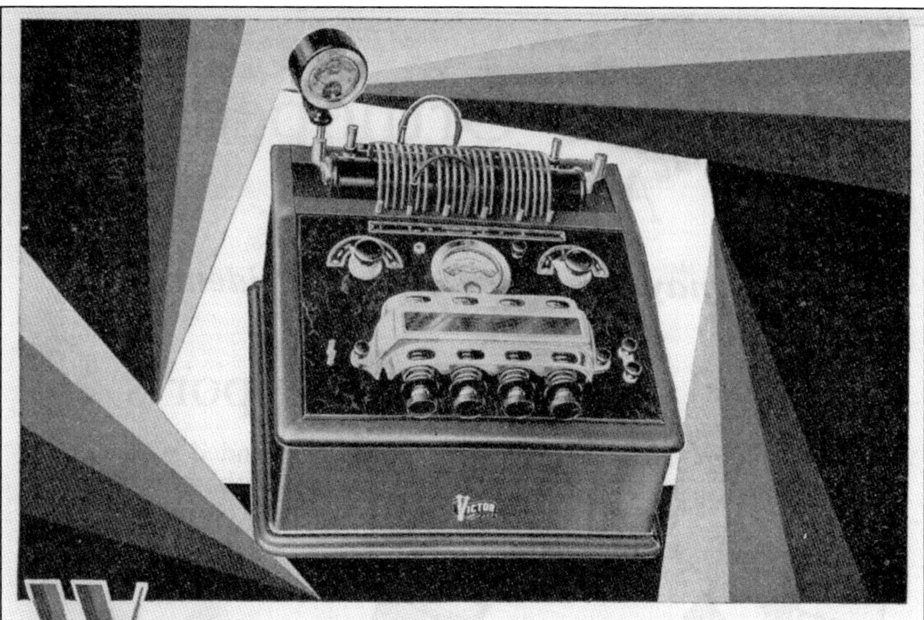

When you want heat deep within the tissues

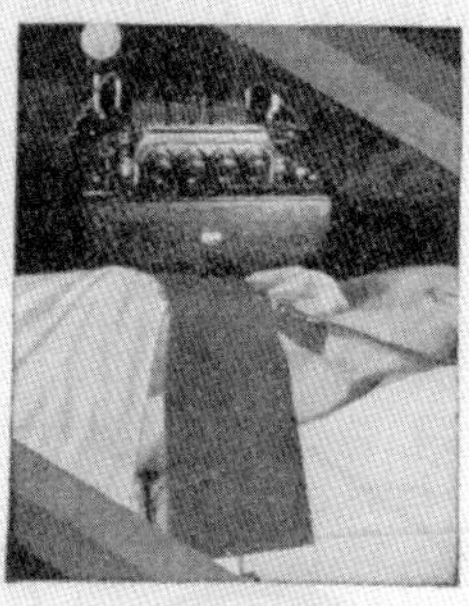

DIATHERMY

According to the definition submitted by the Council on Physical Therapy of the American Medical Association, "Diathermy is a term applied to the use of a high frequency current to generate heat within some part of the body. When such a current is passed through the body at a sufficient voltage and amperage, the resistance offered by the tissues intervening between the electrodes causes heat to be generated in such tissues."

WHERE a deep-seated condition exists, indicating the use of heat as a therapeutic measure, it seems a waste of time to employ a hot water bottle or electric heating pad, when an efficient high-frequency apparatus will produce the desired heat, deep within the tissues, so quickly and thoroughly. No other means is so conveniently available with which to introduce, artificially, heat to any internal part of the body.

With the Victor Vario-Frequency Diathermy apparatus you obtain a quality of current that has the maximum therapeutic effect, and which at the same time is comfortable and within the tolerance of the individual patient. This is because the design of the machine provides a selective range of both voltage and frequency, so that a combination of these two factors may be selected as best suited to the treatment in hand.

Buffalo—1100 Electric Bldg.

PHYSICAL THERAPY DEPARTMENT

VICTOR X-RAY CORPORATION

Manufacturers of the Coolidge Tube and complete line of X-Ray Apparatus — VICTOR — *Physical Therapy Apparatus, Electrocardiographs, and other Specialties*

2012 Jackson Boulevard *Branches in all Principal Cities* **Chicago, Ill., U.S.A.**

A GENERAL ELECTCIC GE **ORGANIZATION**

This May 1929 *Bulletin* advertisement shows the Victor Vario-Frequency Diathermy apparatus. Diathermy applied a high-frequency current to generate heat deep within parts of the body. It was considered an alternative to hot water bottles or electric heating pads at that time.

WOMEN PHYSICIANS ELECTED TO OFFICE

For the first time in the history of the Medical Society of the County of Erie women physicians now hold office in the organization. Dr. Louise W. Beamis for the office of Secretary, and Dr. Mary J. Kazmierczak to represent the Society as one of eight delegates from Erie County to the annual meeting of the State Medical Society, were the choice of a majority of members who voted at the annual election, held December 17, 1928.

The history of medical women in Buffalo and Erie County begins with the admission of Mary Blair Moody to the medical department of

January, 1929 9

the University of Buffalo, in 1874, this being one of the first medical schools to admit women. Dr. Moody was elected to membership in this Society in 1877, and was the first woman to be added to the list of members. She practiced in Buffalo several years, subsequently moved to New Haven, Conn., and died in California in 1919.

Dr. Moody had an immediate successor in the college halls in the person of Mary Berkes, who matriculated in 1877, and was graduated in medicine in 1880. In 1886 Dr. Berkes married Dr. Samuel W. Wetmore. Dr. Mary Berkes Wetmore died in Buffalo in 1928.

Since the medical department of the University of Buffalo first admitted women, 142 have received diplomas, many of them with high honors.

In 1892 the trustees of Niagara University voted to admit women to the medical department of that institution. Anna Earl Hutchinson of North Evans was the first woman to avail herself of that privilege. She was graduated in 1895. Mary O'Malley of Barker, N. Y., was graduated in medicine from Niagara University in 1897, a year before that medical school was amalgamated with the University of Buffalo.

This 1929 *Bulletin* article marks the first time in Medical Society history that women physicians held office in the organization. Dr. Louise Beamis was installed as secretary, and Dr. Mary Kazmierczak was selected as one of eight delegates from Erie County at the state medical society's annual meeting.

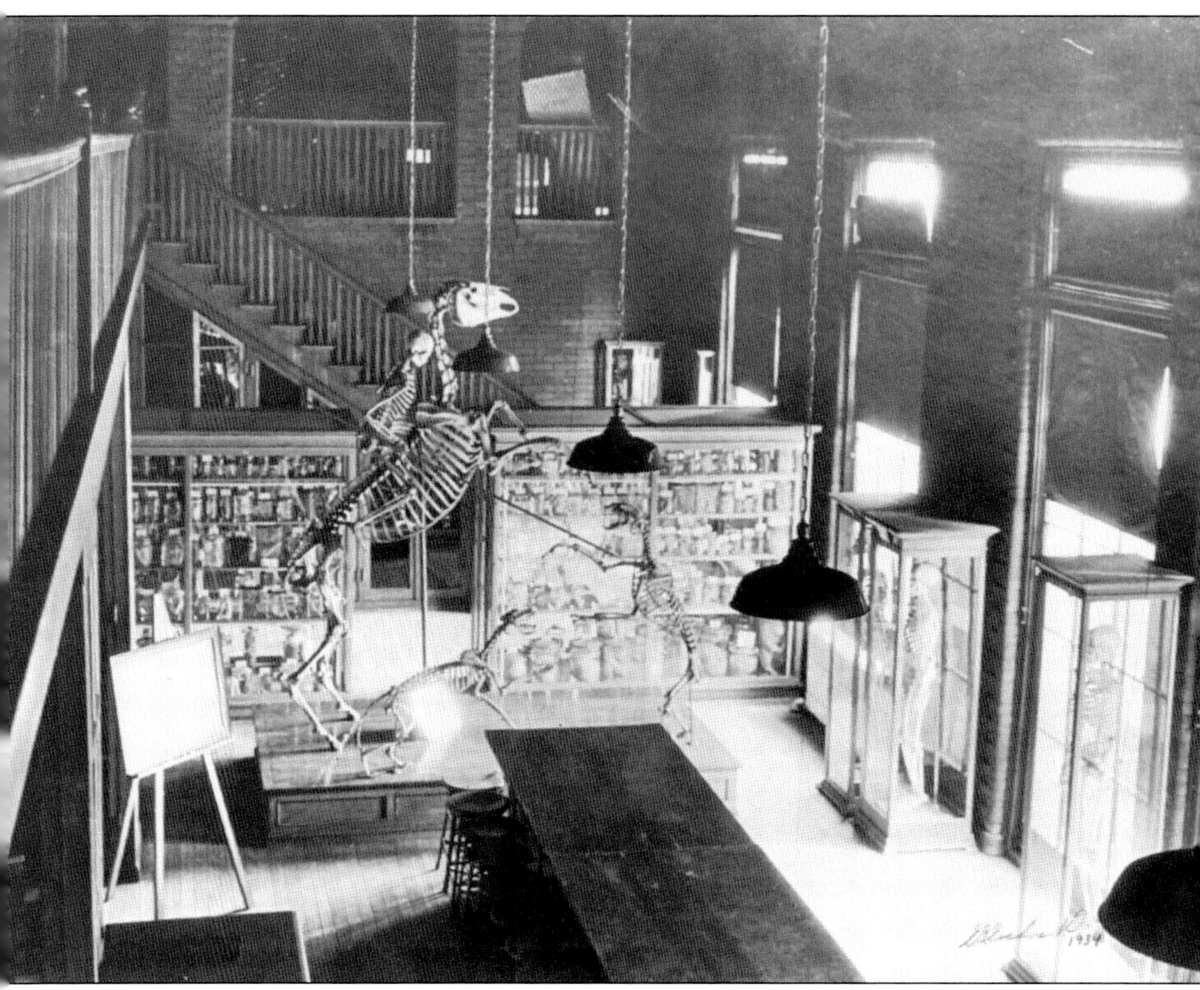

This 1934 image shows the interior of the Pathology Museum in the old University of Buffalo School of Medicine building. It was not until 1953, when Capen Hall opened, that the School of Medicine moved to the Main Street campus. (Courtesy of University Archives, University at Buffalo.)

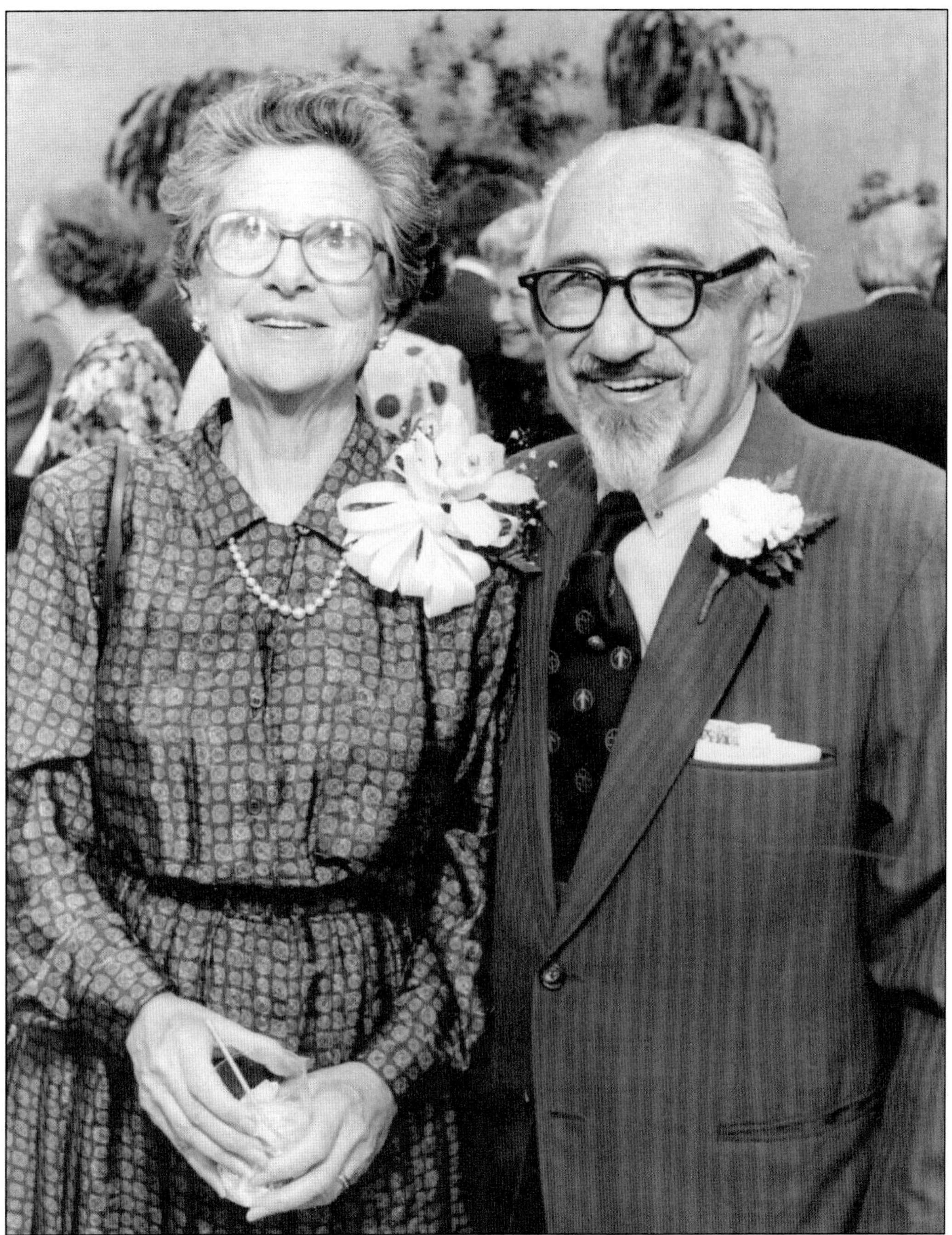

Dr. Robert Warner, a Medical Society of Erie County member, shown here with his wife, was an internationally prominent pediatrician who helped develop a simple test for genetic birth defects. Dr. Warner was well regarded for his role in assisting Dr. Robert Guthrie in the development of the phenylketonuria (PKU) test. Dr. Warner graduated from Harvard College in 1935 and earned his medical degree from the University of Chicago in 1939. He practiced at Children's Hospital, received the Pediatrician of the Year award from the Buffalo Pediatric Society, and served as associate professor of pediatrics at the University at Buffalo School of Medicine.

STRAPPED FOR RICKETS

The swaddled infant pictured at right is one of the famous works in terra cotta exquisitely modeled by the fifteenth century Italian sculptor, Andrea della Robbia. In that day infants were bandaged from birth to preserve the symmetry of their bodies, but still the gibbous spine and distorted limbs of severe rickets often made their appearance.

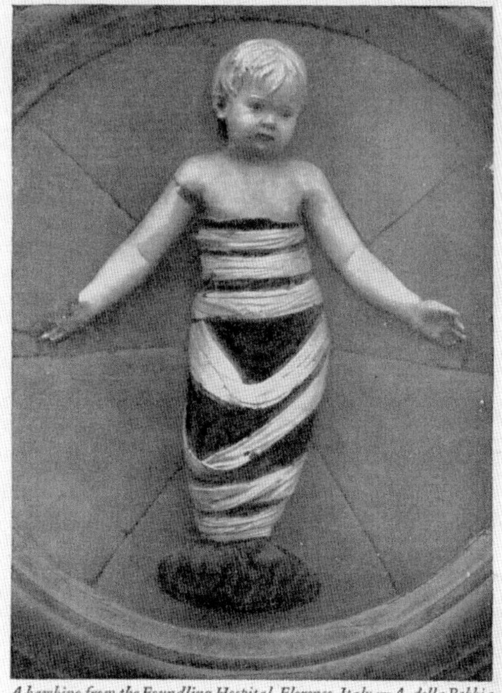

A bambino from the Foundling Hospital, Florence, Italy,—A. della Robbia

SWADDLING was practised down through the centuries, from Biblical times to Glisson's day, in the vain hope that it would prevent the deformities of rickets. Even in sunny Italy swaddling was a prevailing custom, recommended by that early pediatrician, Soranus of Ephesus, who discoursed on "Why the Majority of Roman Children are Distorted."

"This is observed to happen more in the neighborhood of Rome than in other places," he wrote. "If no one oversees the infant's movements, his limbs do in the generality of cases become twisted. . . . Hence, when he first begins to sit he must be propped by swathings of bandages. . . ." Hundreds of years later swaddling was still prevalent in Italy, as attested by the sculptures of the della Robbias and their contemporaries. For infants who were strong Glisson suggested placing "Leaden Shooes" on their feet and suspending them with swaddling bands in mid-air.

How amazed the ancients would have been to know that bones can be helped to grow straight simply by internal administration of a few drops of Oleum Percomorphum. What to them would have been a miracle has become a commonplace of science. Because it can be administered in drop dosage, Oleum Percomorphum is especially suitable for young and premature infants, who are most susceptible to rickets. Its vitamins A and D derived from natural sources, this product has 100 times the potency of cod liver oil.* Important also to your patients, Oleum Percomorphum is an an economical antiricketic.

Oleum Percomorphum offers not less than 60,000 U.S.P. vitamin A units and 8,500 U.S.P. vitamin D units per gram. Supplied in 10 and 50 c.c. bottles, also in boxes of 25 and 100 ten-drop soluble gelatin capsules containing not less than 13,300 vitamin A units and 1,850 vitamin D units (equal to more than 5 teaspoonfuls of cod liver oil*).

*U.S.P. Minimum Standard

MEAD JOHNSON & COMPANY
EVANSVILLE, INDIANA, U. S. A.

Please enclose professional card when requesting samples of Mead Johnson products to cooperate in preventing their reaching unauthorized persons.

Found in the January 1938 *Bulletin* was this advertisement for the drop dosage drug Oleum Percomorphum, which was used to treat infants born with rickets. At the time, Oleum Percomorphum was marketed as offering concentrated units of Vitamins A and D and was touted as having "100 times the potency of cod liver oil."

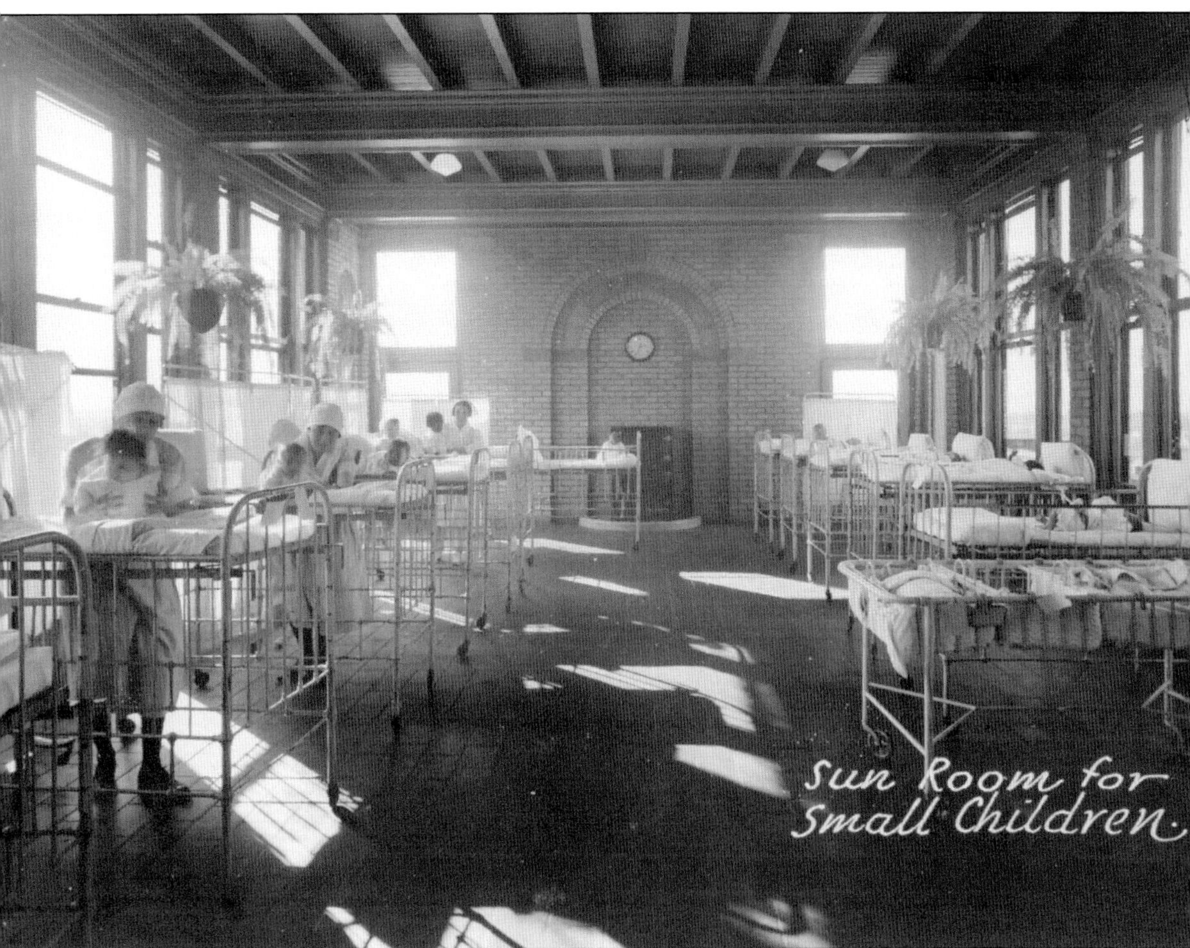

Pictured here is a sunroom for small children at E.J. Meyer Memorial Hospital. Its founder, Dr. Edward J. Meyer, was largely responsible for Buffalo City Hospital's affiliation with the University of Buffalo. Dedication ceremonies for the new Meyer Hospital were held on April 20, 1939 (four years after Dr. Meyer's death in 1935), under the joint auspices of the Medical Society of Erie County, the Buffalo Academy of Medicine, and the hospital staff. (Courtesy of University Archives, University at Buffalo.)

GROUP*

MALPRACTICE INSURANCE

Medical Society of the State of New York

•

H. F. WANVIG

Insurance Representative

70 PINE STREET NEW YORK CITY

•

Erie County Representative

ALBERT DODGE, INC.

CL. 4264

321 Genesee Building

BUFFALO, N. Y.

**For Members of the Society Only*

AT J. N. ADAM'S

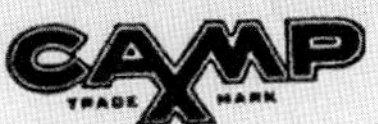

SURGICAL GARMENTS

for Maternity
Post-Natal
Post-operative
and Sacro-Iliac cases

are expertly fitted by corsetieres who are graduates of the Camp School of Surgical Fitters. Your prescription is filled promptly and exactly.

J. N. ADAM & CO.

Camp Garments — Corset Shop

THIRD FLOOR

ABDOMINAL or POST OPERATIVE SUPPORTS--New Type Sacro Belts

to meet your most exacting requirements. Experience gained in many thousands of cases has enabled Rice designers to produce garments to correctly meet most every conceivable need. The new type "ring-pull" Sacro Belt, while very light and comfortable, furnishes unusual support and is highly effective. You, as a physician, will appreciate "the difference" the minute you see them. Our designers and men and women fitting experts are at your service. May we work with you?

WILLIAM S. RICE, INC.

168 FRANKLIN ST.
Near Statler Hotel

BUFFALO, NEW YORK

Phone
MAdison 2730

SPECIAL HEALTH AND ACCIDENT POLICY

Sponsored By

ERIE COUNTY MEDICAL SOCIETY

(For Members Only)

CHARLES J. SELLERS, Agent

1617 LIBERTY BANK BLDG. WASH. 1930

These advertisements in the April 1941 *Bulletin* include one from long standing Medical Society partner Charles J. Sellers of Charles J. Sellers & Co. Inc. offering special health and accident policies for physician members.

MEDICAL SOCIETY, COUNTY OF ERIE

FALL CLINICAL DAY AND FIFTY YEAR DINNER

Thursday, November 13, 1941
Hotel Statler, Buffalo

To Honor Physicians Who Have Practiced Fifty Years or More

CLINICAL SESSIONS – TERRACE ROOM – 3 to 5 P.M

JENNINGS C. LITZENBERG, M.D., Minneapolis
"FIFTY YEARS OF CHANGE IN OBSTETRICS"

JONATHAN C. MEAKINS, M.D., Montreal
"THE HEART FROM THE STANDPOINT OF THE GENERAL PRACTITIONER"

CHARLES GORDON HEYD, M.D., New York City
"THE CONCEPT OF LIVER DEATHS"

"GET ACQUAINTED HOUR" – CHINESE ROOM – 5 P.M.

DINNER -- BALL ROOM -- 7 P.M.

. . . Speaker . . .
LOGAN CLENDENNING, M.D., Kansas City
"RESISTANCE TO CHANGE AS A FACTOR IN MEDICAL PROGRESS"

The October 1941 *Bulletin* advertised a celebration at the Hotel Statler of the Medical Society's 50th year, at which time physicians who practiced regionally for 50 years or more would be honored.

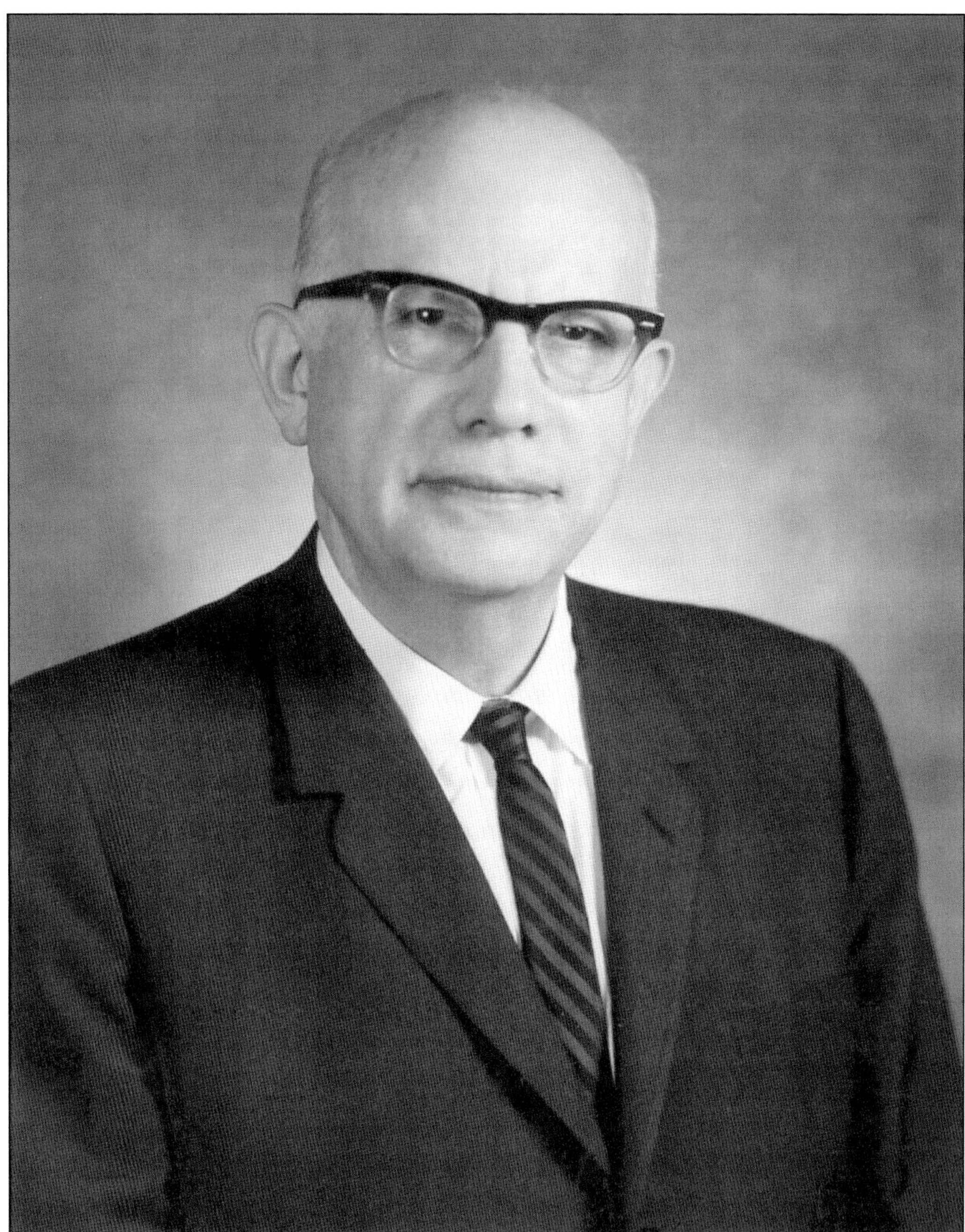

Buffalo physician Ernest Witebsky, MD, attended medical school at the University of Frankfurt in 1926 before he was expelled from Germany by the Nazi regime. Dr. Witebsky worked at the University of Geneva in Switzerland and New York City's Mount Sinai Hospital before joining Buffalo's School of Medicine faculty in 1936. From 1941 to 1967, Dr. Witebsky was professor and head of the Department of Bacteriology and Immunology, publishing more than 300 scientific papers. The last tribute to Dr. Witebsky was in June 1968 when he was officially inaugurated by the International Convocation on Immunology for his contribution as a renowned immunologist in the United States. (Courtesy of University Archives, University at Buffalo.)

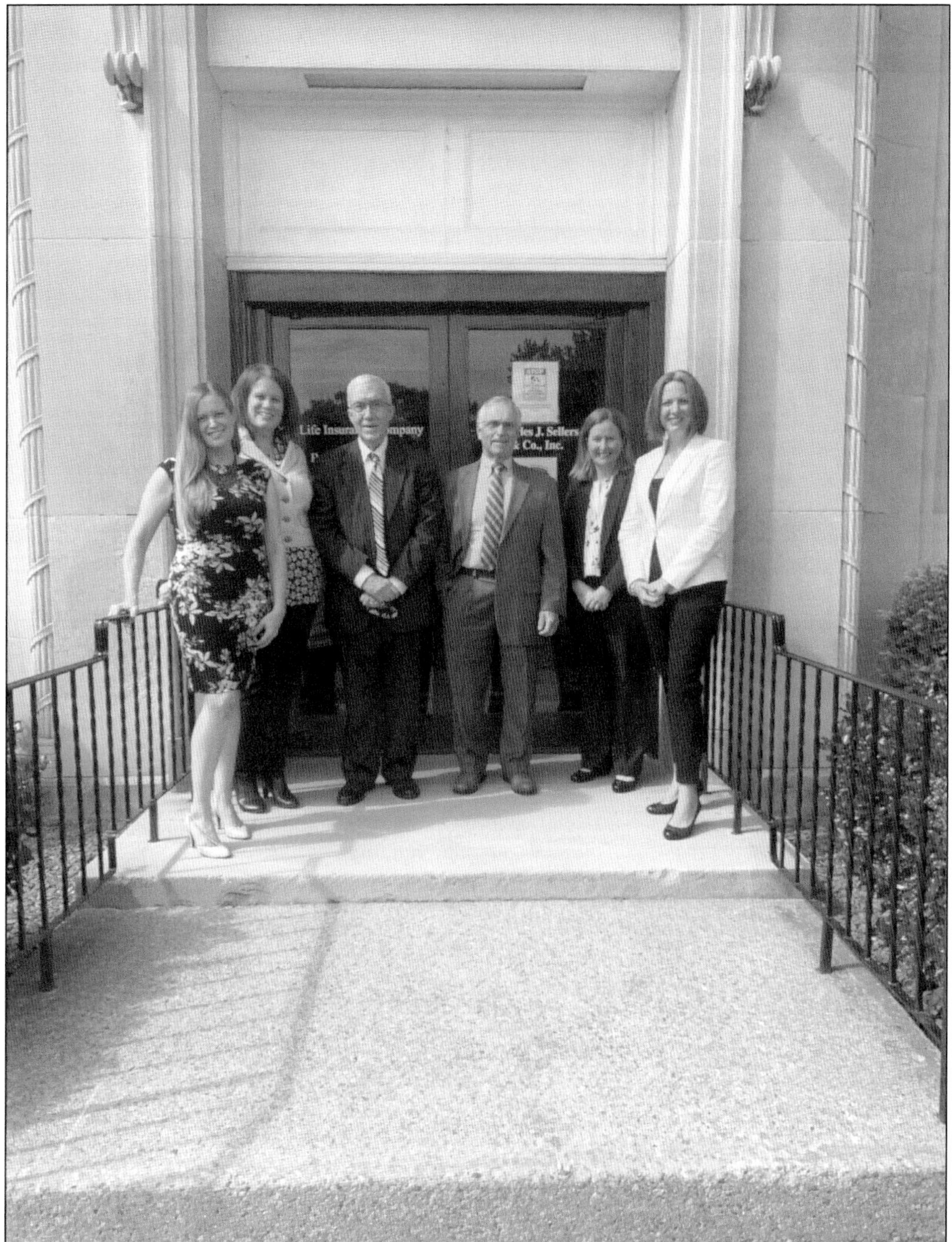

The Medical Society of Erie County first endorsed Charles J. Sellers & Co.'s disability policy for members on March 17, 1941. In the 80 years since, the firm has written all types of insurance for thousands of members, helping themselves, their families, and their practices through life's unexpected events. Pictured are, from left to right, Ann Sellers, Amy Burnett, Tom Sellers, Charlie Sellers, Kate Sellers, and Ellen Behm.

10 BULLETIN March, 1942

part of the Office for Emergency Management which in turn is part of the Executive Office of the President. The director of the ODHWS is Paul V. McNutt, who is also Federal Security Administrator.

WOMAN'S AUXILIARY

Dr. W. W. Bauer of Chicago, Ill., Director of the Bureau of Health Education of the American Medical Association, will address a public luncheon meeting at the Hotel Statler on April 13th. Dr. Bauer's appearance will be sponsored jointly by the Medical Societies of Erie and Niagara Counties. The Woman's Auxiliary, with Mrs. John C. Brady as chairman, is in charge of arrangements for the day.

AUXILIARY'S PART IN NATIONAL DEFENSE

Members of the Woman's Auxiliary will dress in uniforms representing the various fields in national defense at the next monthly meeting to be held Tuesday, March 31st, Chinese Room of the Hotel Statler. Mrs. Franklin C. Southworth will be chairman for the day.

MRS. JOSEPH C. SCANIO,
Chairman of Publicity.

DON'T FORGET THE DATE!

Wistaria Ball

SATURDAY EVENING, APRIL 11th

Tickets $1.10, Tax Included

Hotel Statler — Ballroom

CREDITORS COMMERCIAL CORPORATION
An Ethical, Conservative Collection Service
... FOR DOCTORS ONLY ...
Established 1913 971-973 Ellicott Square MAdison 3013-3014

The March 1942 *Bulletin* included a reminder to members to save the date for the highly regarded Wistaria Ball. The ball was to take place at the prestigious Hotel Statler ballroom on the evening of Saturday, April 11, 1942, with tickets priced at $1.10 per person.

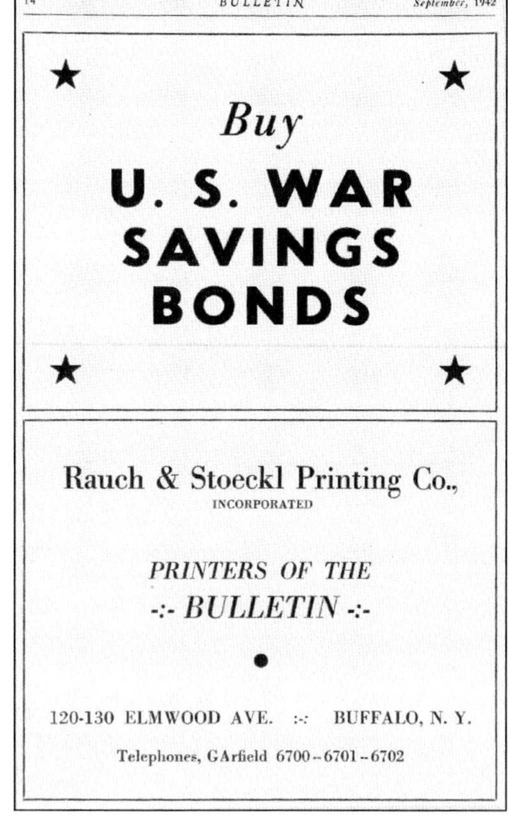

14 BULLETIN September, 1942

★ ★

Buy

U. S. WAR SAVINGS BONDS

★ ★

Rauch & Stoeckl Printing Co.,
INCORPORATED

PRINTERS OF THE
-:- BULLETIN -:-

•

120-130 ELMWOOD AVE. :-: BUFFALO, N. Y.

Telephones, GArfield 6700 - 6701 - 6702

This advertisement in a 1942 *Bulletin* urged members to support the war effort by purchasing war savings bonds. The Series E bonds had a minimum maturity period of 10 years and were sold at 75 percent of face value with a 2.9 percent interest rate, compounded semiannually.

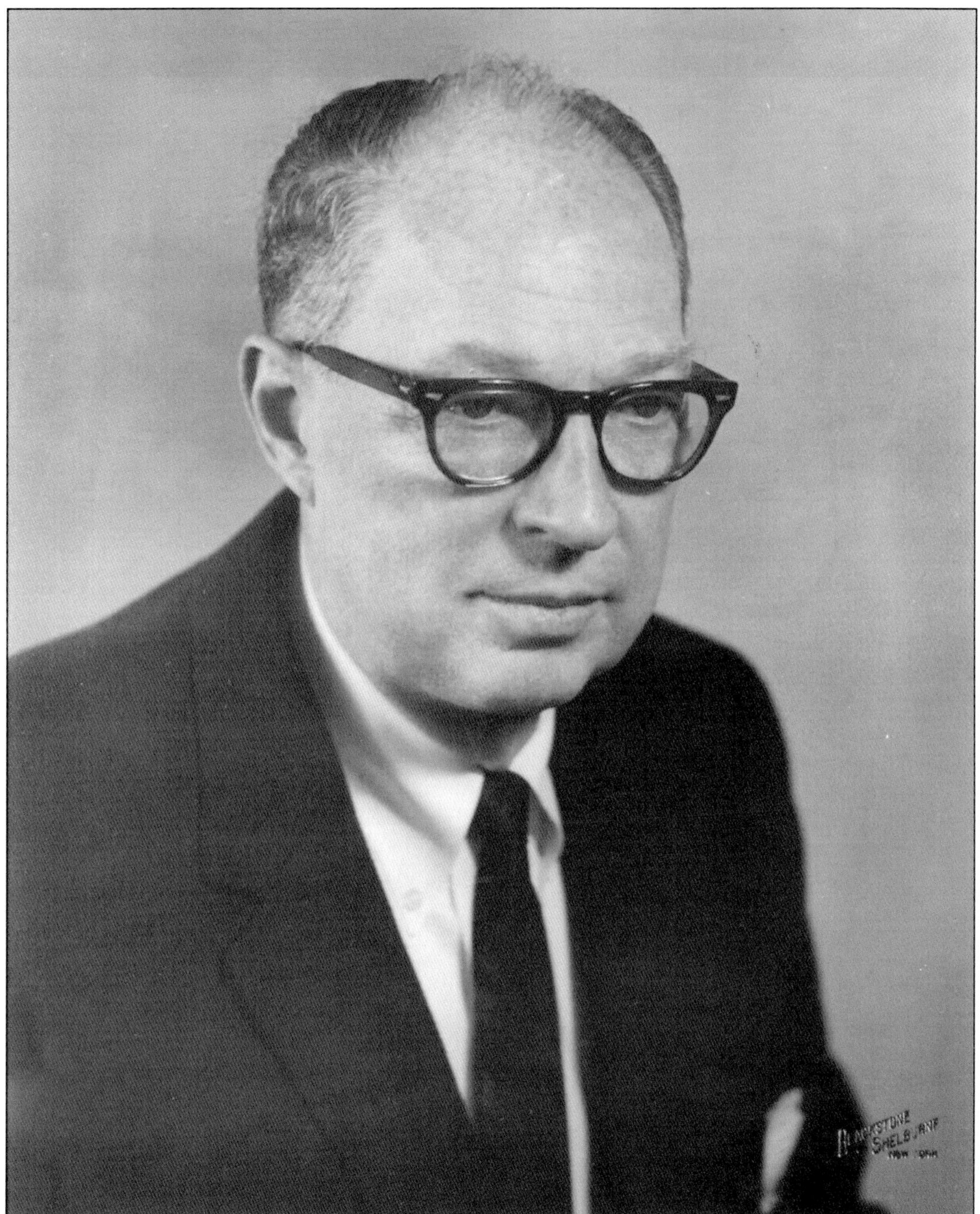

Former Erie County physician Dr. Joseph Godfrey, a south Buffalo native, became one of the most respected and successful physicians in the United States. He served as physician-surgeon for the Buffalo Bills of the American and National Football Leagues from 1947 to 1978. Dr. Godfrey was named "Mr. Sports Machine" by the American Orthopedics Society for Sports Medicine in 1977. (Courtesy of University Archives, University at Buffalo.)

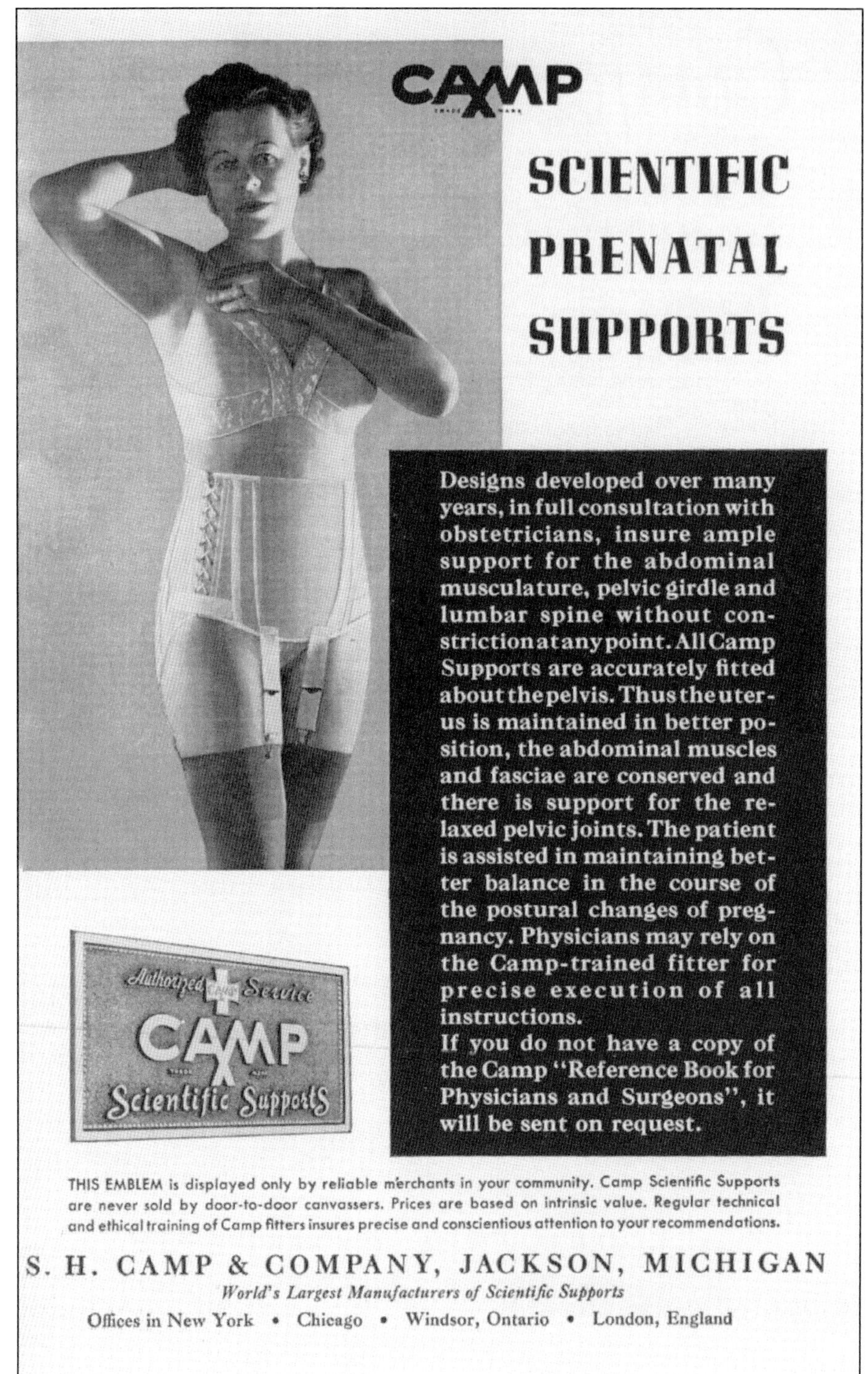

This 1949 *Bulletin* advertisement was for a scientific prenatal support pelvic girdle manufactured by Camp Scientific Supports. It was designed to help women maintain better balance due to postural changes throughout the course of their pregnancy.

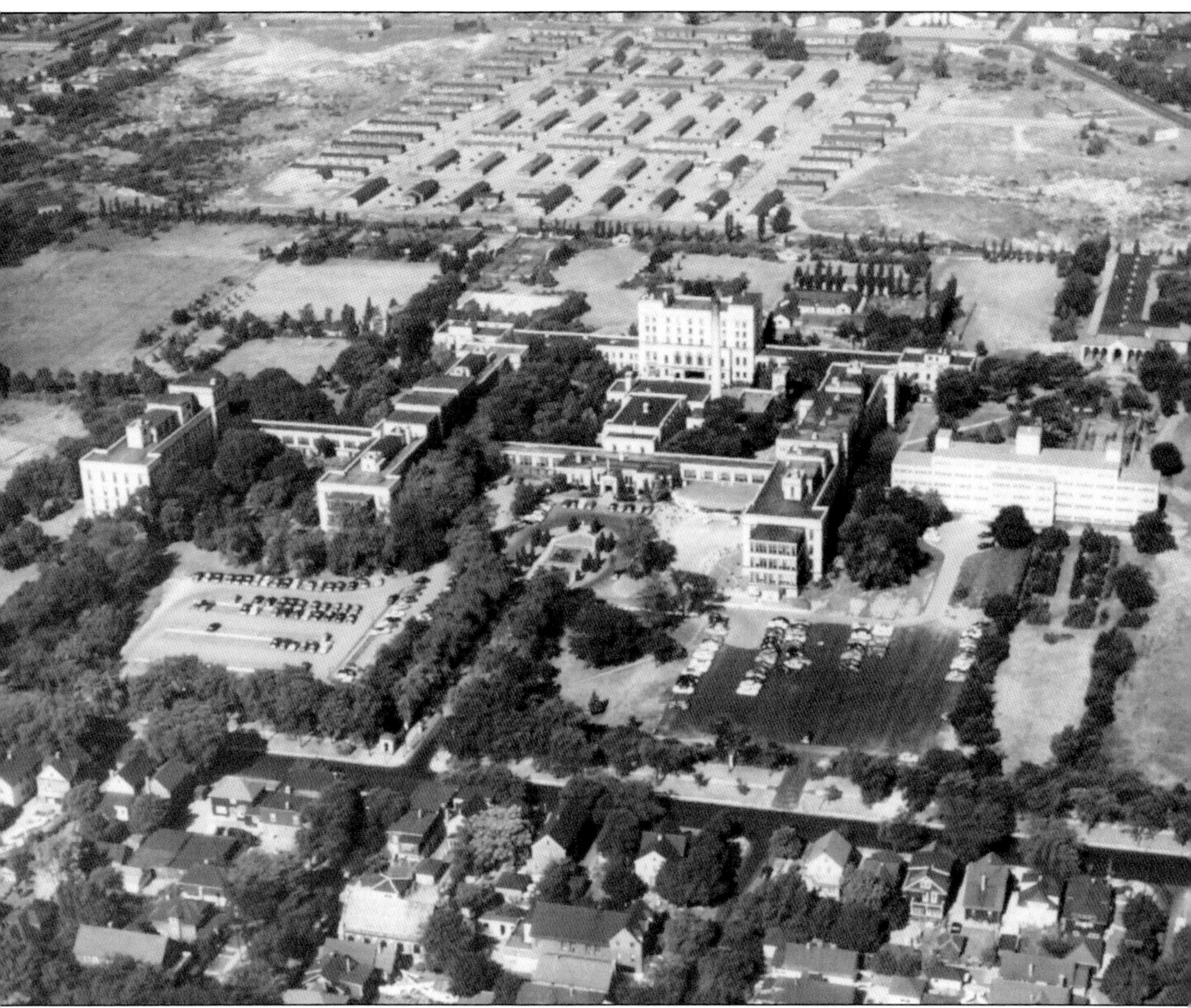

E.J. Meyer Memorial Hospital is pictured here in 1950; it is currently known as the Erie County Medical Center. The hospital was originally named after Dr. Edward J. Meyer in 1939. He served as the first president of the Buffalo City Hospital Board of Managers and guided the hospital through nearly two decades until his death in 1935. In addition to his remarkable career at Buffalo City Hospital, Dr. Meyer was also a member of the faculty at the University of Buffalo, where he received his medical degree in 1891. (Courtesy of University Archives, University at Buffalo.)

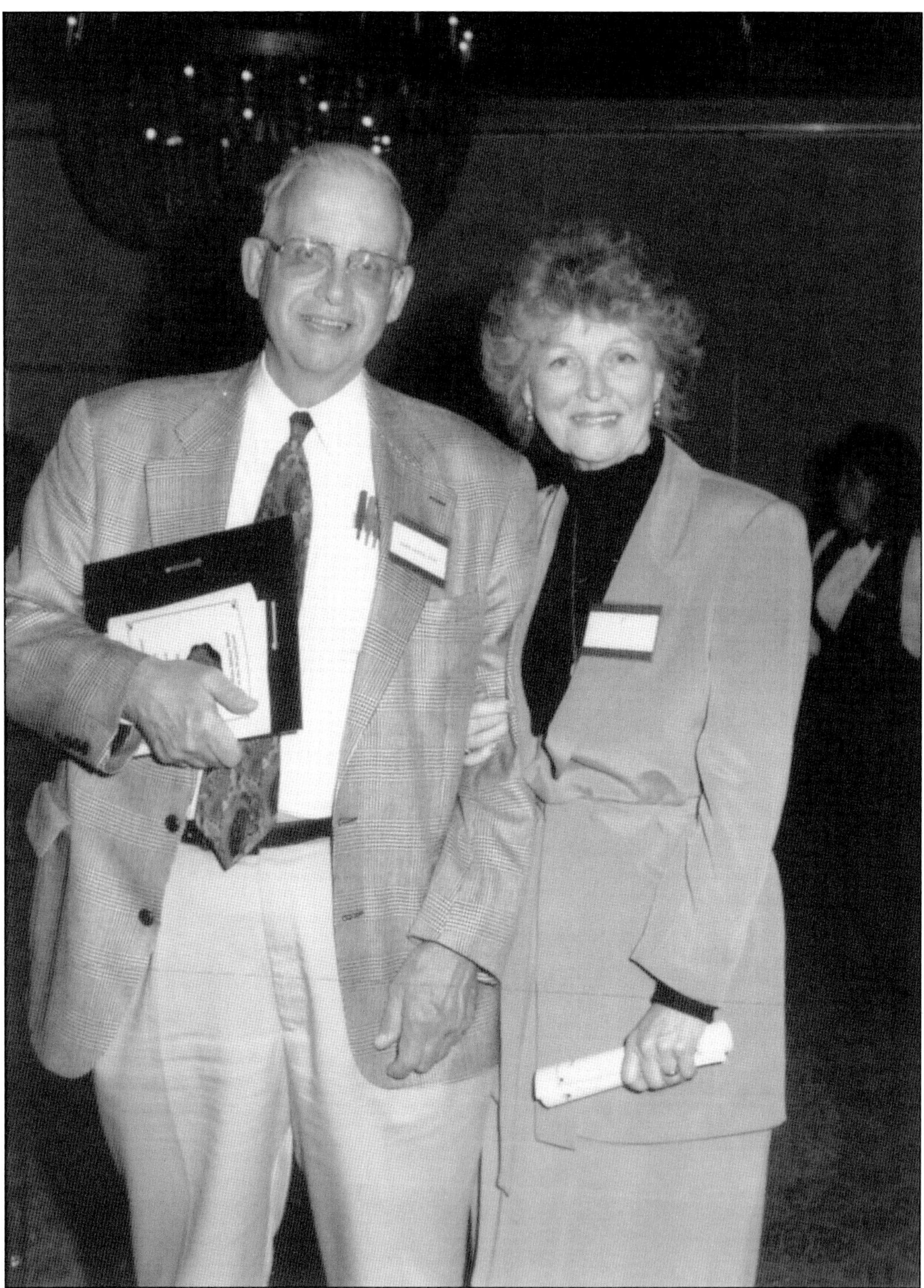

Pictured here with his wife, Joan, is Medical Society member Dr. John Bozer, a renowned cardiologist and former medical director of the Cardiac Rehabilitation Program at Buffalo General Hospital. Born in Buffalo, Dr. Bozer earned a bachelor's degree with honors from Harvard University in 1948 and graduated from the College of Physicians and Surgeons of Columbia College in 1952.

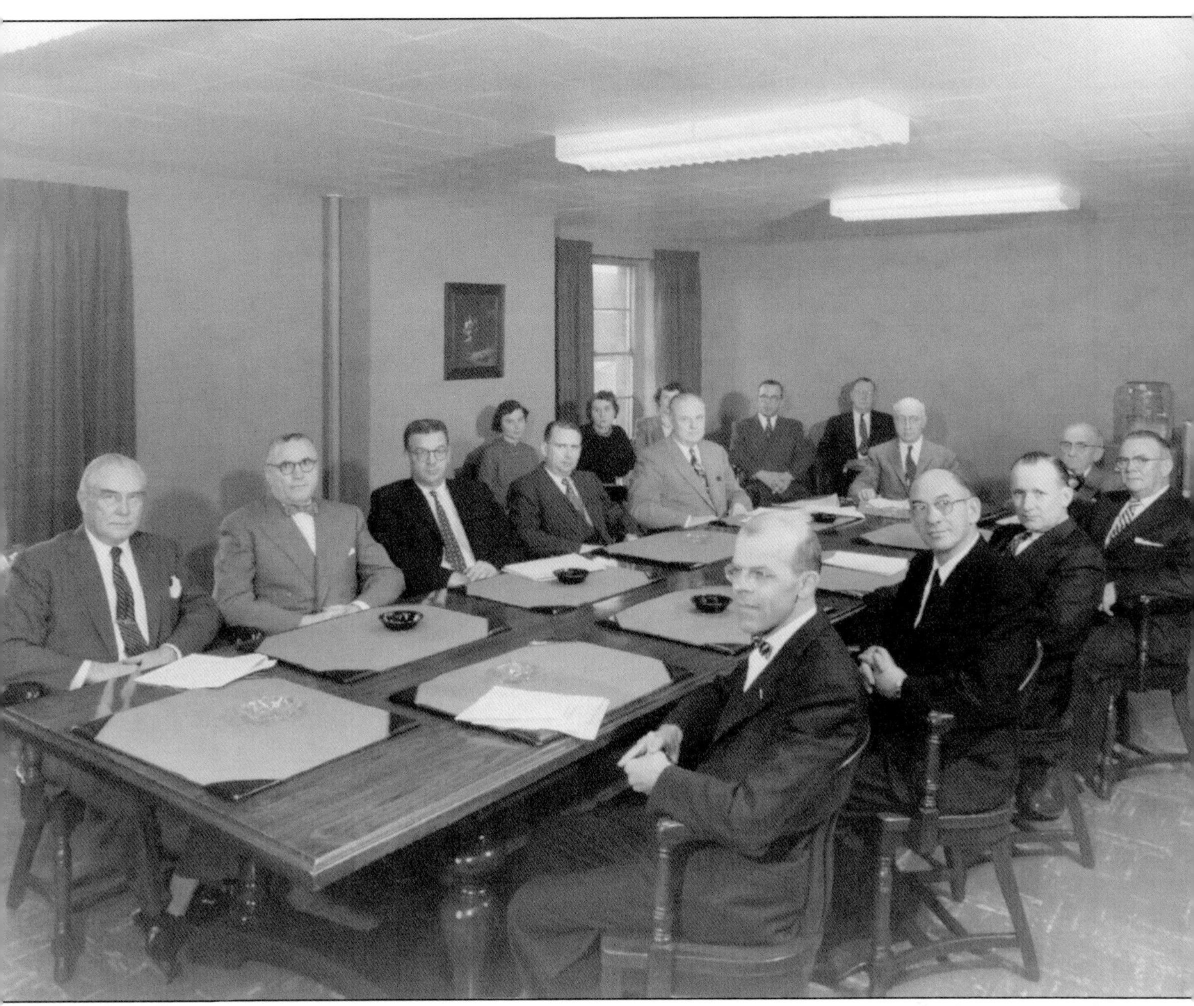

This photograph shows the new Medical Society of Erie County comitia minora as they convened for their first meeting of the year on January 17, 1956, in the new offices of the society on the second floor of the Hotel Statler. Seated at the head of the table is Matthew Callanan, MD, the president at the time.

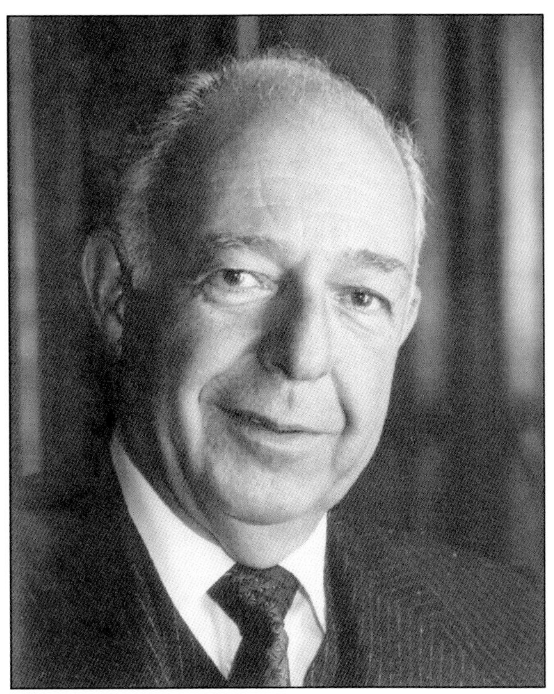

Dr. Pasquale Greco was an accomplished surgeon and urologist and the past president of the medical staff at Millard Fillmore Hospital from 1953 to 1982. Dr. Greco was affiliated with every major hospital in the Buffalo region, including Roswell Park Memorial Institute, Buffalo Children's, Buffalo General, Erie County Medical Center, Kenmore Mercy, and Sister's Hospital.

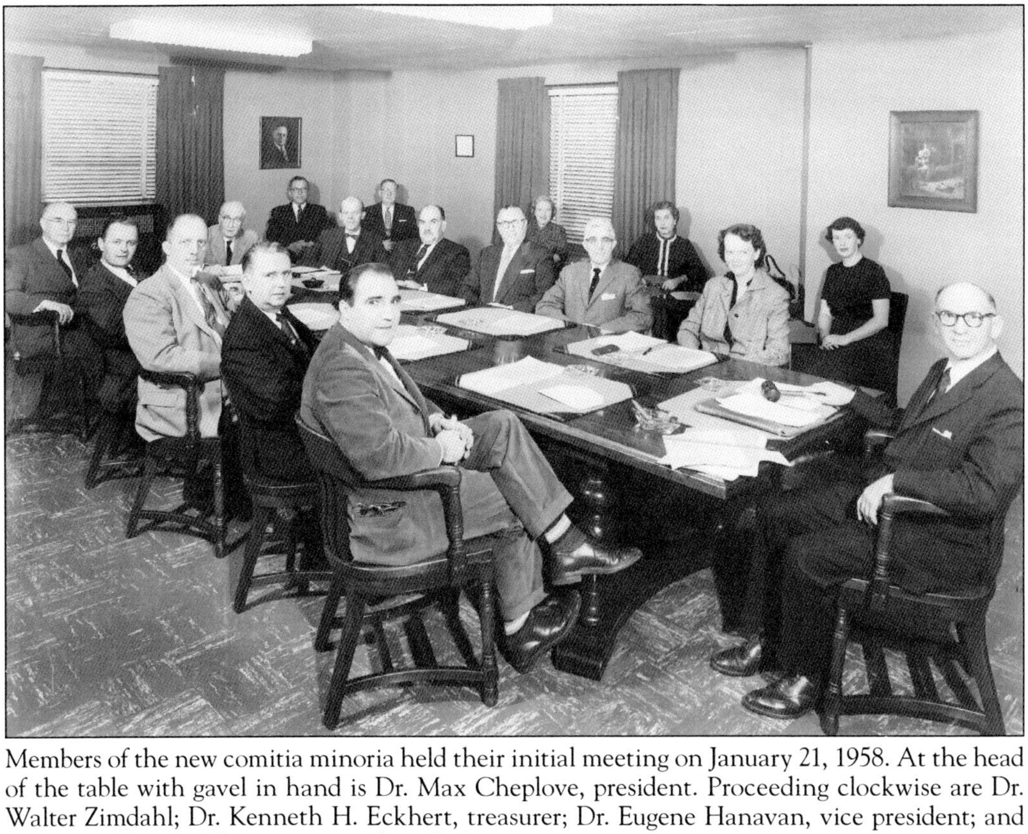

Members of the new comitia minoria held their initial meeting on January 21, 1958. At the head of the table with gavel in hand is Dr. Max Cheplove, president. Proceeding clockwise are Dr. Walter Zimdahl; Dr. Kenneth H. Eckhert, treasurer; Dr. Eugene Hanavan, vice president; and George Collins Jr. The rest are unidentified.

Five

The 1960s

In 1967, Buffalo was the location of one of the 159 race riots that took place across the United States. The long, hot summer saw riots in the cities of Atlanta, Boston, Cincinnati, Tampa, and Buffalo in June. The riots extended to Detroit, Birmingham, Chicago, New York City, Milwaukee, Minneapolis, New Britain, Rochester, Plainfield, and Toledo in July.

The Buffalo riot took place on the east side of Buffalo from June 26 to July 1, 1967. The riots shut down the city and resulted in over 40 people being injured and 14 suffering gunshot wounds. The nation saw a grim total of 83 dead, thousands injured, and tens of millions of dollars in property destroyed during the riots and the burning of entire neighborhoods to the ground.

The riots began as a response to unemployment, abusive policing, and poor housing within certain areas in the United States. These riots peaked during the summer months when living conditions worsened due to the oppressive heat.

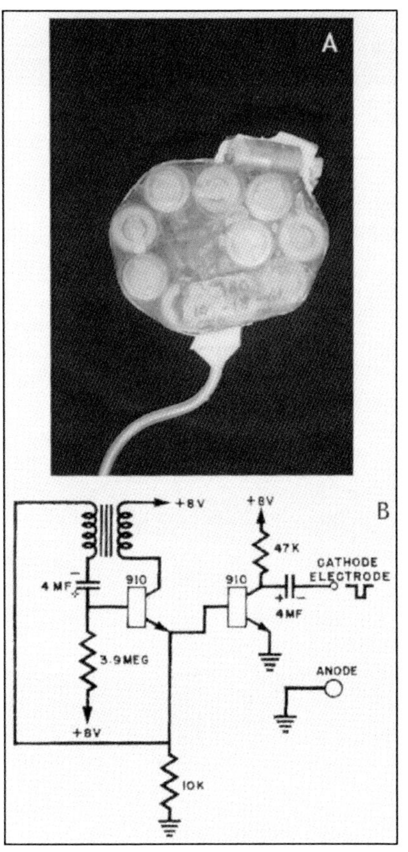

Pictured here is the first-ever pacemaker developed in 1960 by chief of surgery at the Buffalo VA Hospital, Dr. William Chardack. Dr. Chardack invented a pocket-sized pacemaker device designed to deliver regular shocks to a diseased heart, forcing the heart muscles to contract and pump blood throughout the body. (Courtesy of University Archives, University at Buffalo.)

SURGERY

VOL. 48 OCTOBER, 1960 No. 4

Original Communications

A TRANSISTORIZED, SELF-CONTAINED, IMPLANTABLE PACEMAKER FOR THE LONG-TERM CORRECTION OF COMPLETE HEART BLOCK

WILLIAM M. CHARDACK, M.D., ANDREW A. GAGE, M.D., AND WILSON GREATBATCH, M.S., BUFFALO, N. Y.

(From the Surgical Service, Buffalo Veterans Administration Hospital, and the Department of Surgery, University of Buffalo School of Medicine)

A *Bulletin* article from October 1960 featured the first "transistorized, self-contained, implantable pacemaker for the long-term correction of complete heart block." The pacemaker was invented by Dr. William Chardack along with Dr. Andrew Gage, professor emeritus of surgery at the University of Buffalo, and Wilson Greatbatch.

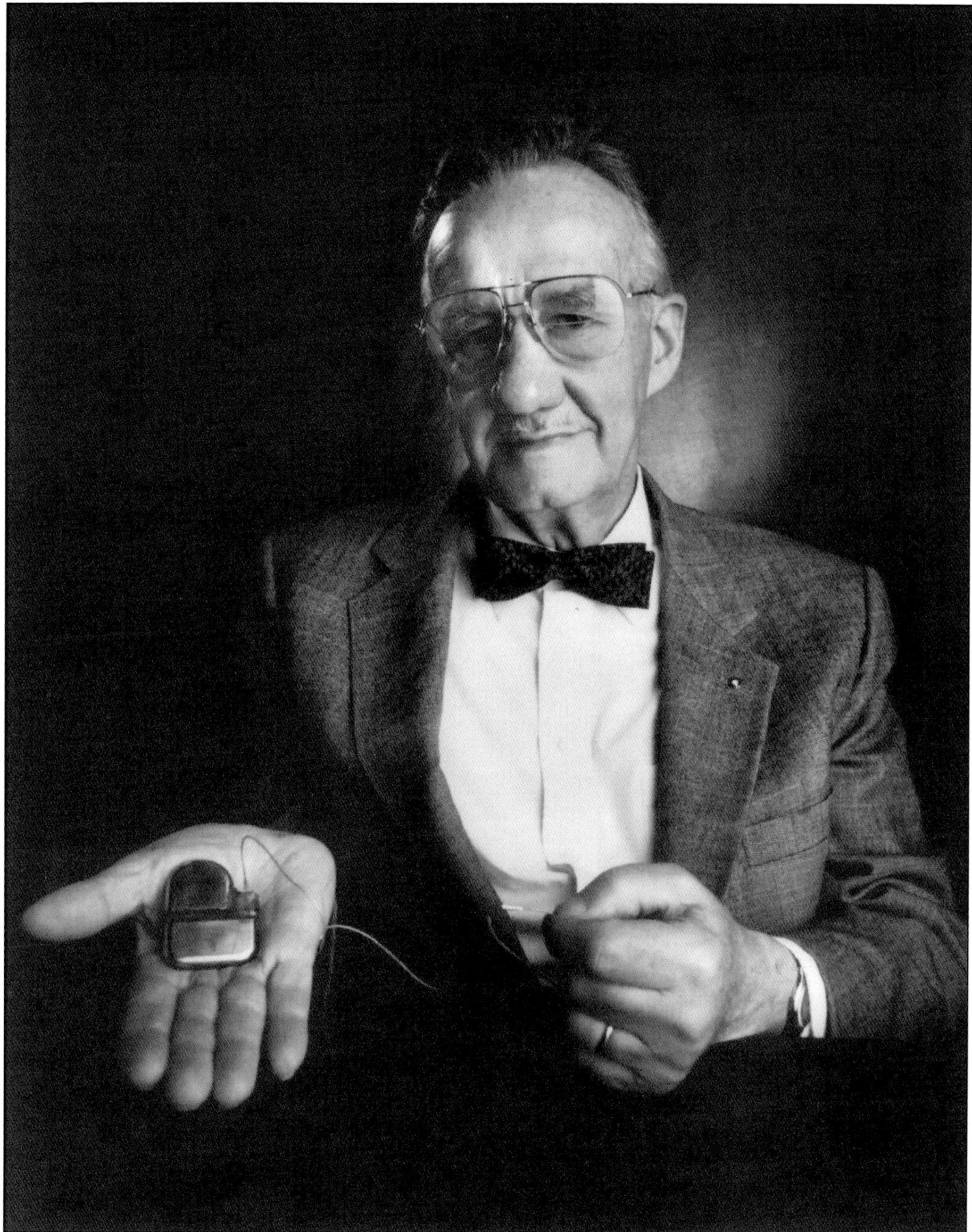

Wilson Greatbatch, an electrical engineer, coinvented with Dr. William Chardack, chief of surgery at Buffalo VA Hospital, the first successful human cardiac pacemaker. Dr. Chardack's pacemaker was first implanted in a patient in the United States on June 6, 1960. (Courtesy of University Archives, University at Buffalo.)

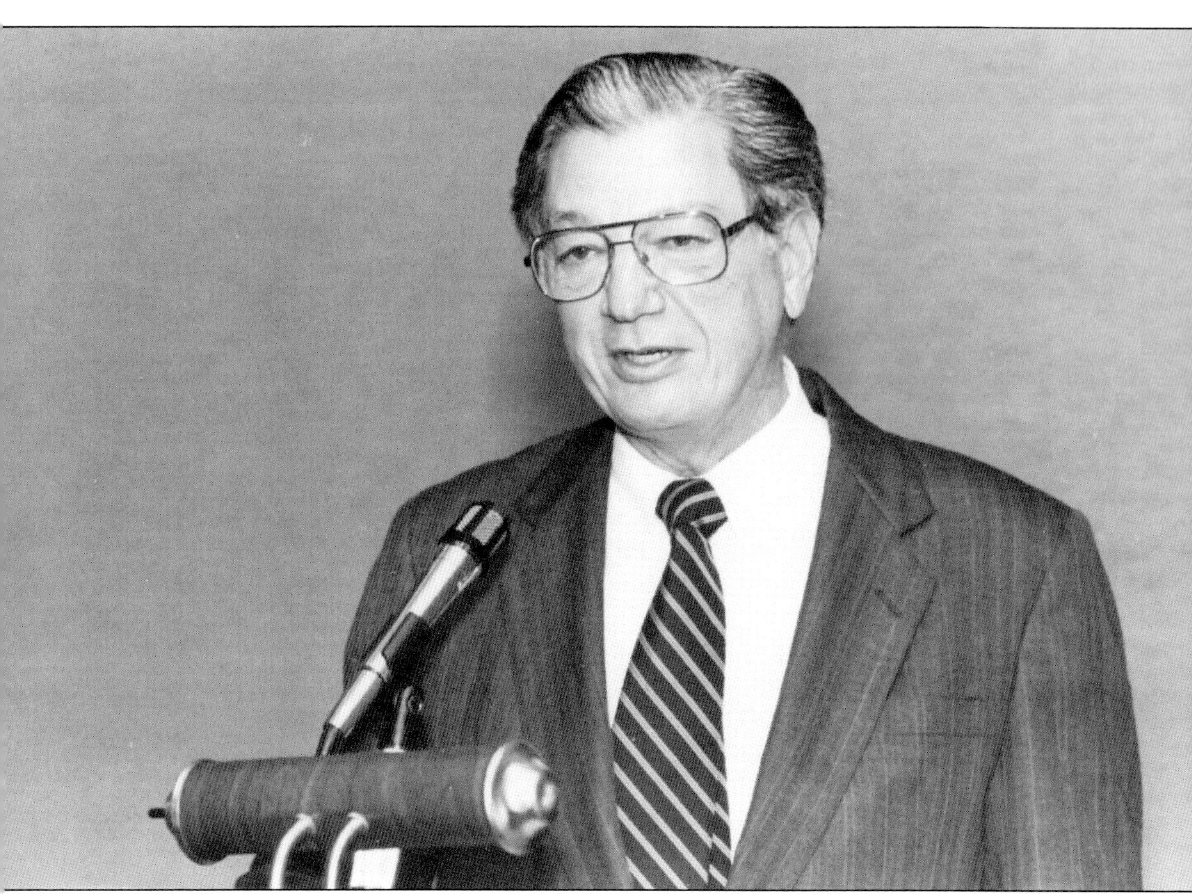

Shown here is Richard Trecasse, executive director of the Medical Society of Erie County from 1963 to 1990. Prior to joining the society, Trecasse served as assistant executive director of the Dade County Medical Society for six years. He died on February 4, 2018.

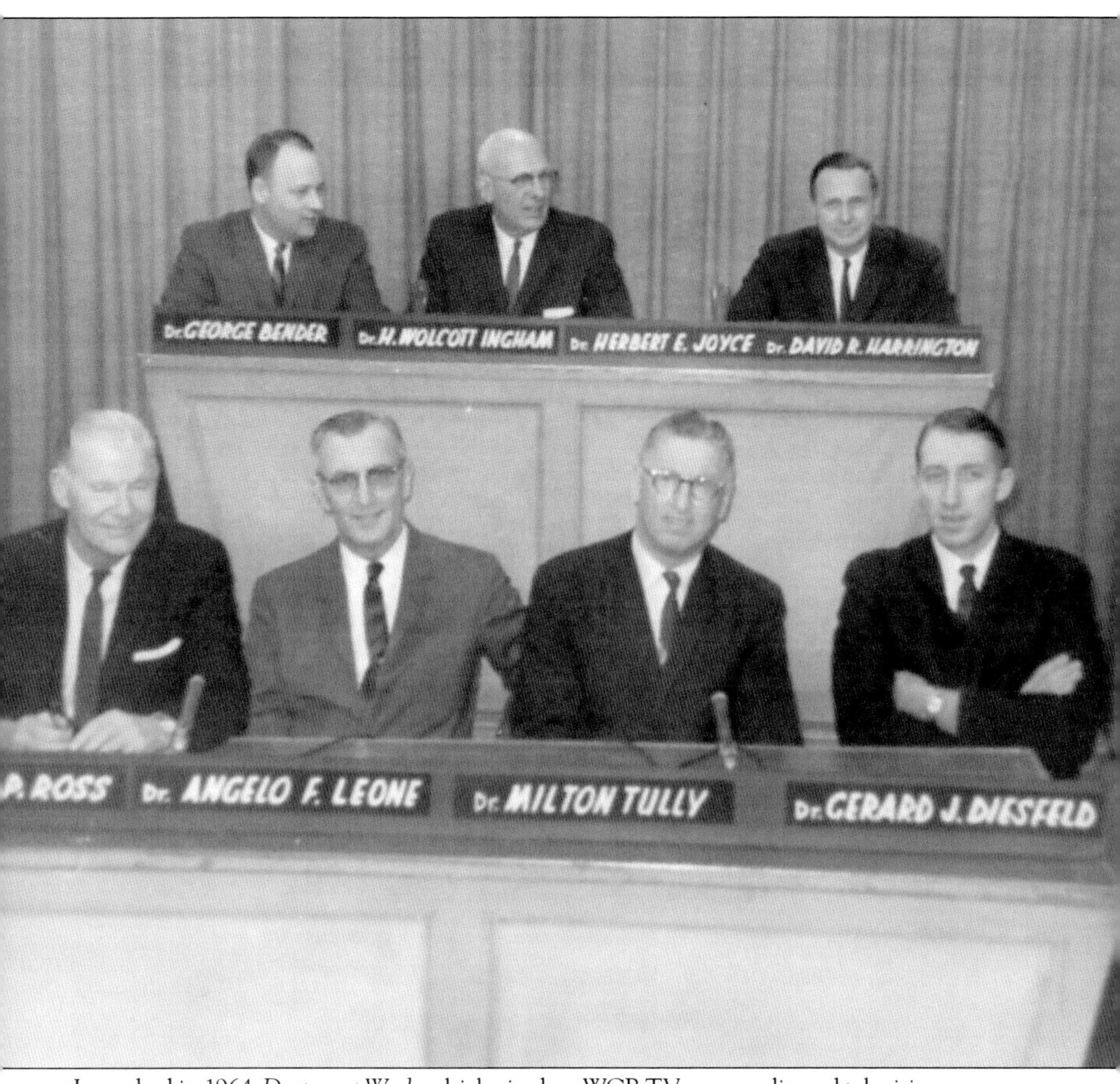

Launched in 1964, *Doctors at Work*, which aired on WGR-TV, was a radio and television program dedicated to public health. *Doctors at Work* was a cooperative effort among six western New York medical societies to present a series of health information programs to the community.

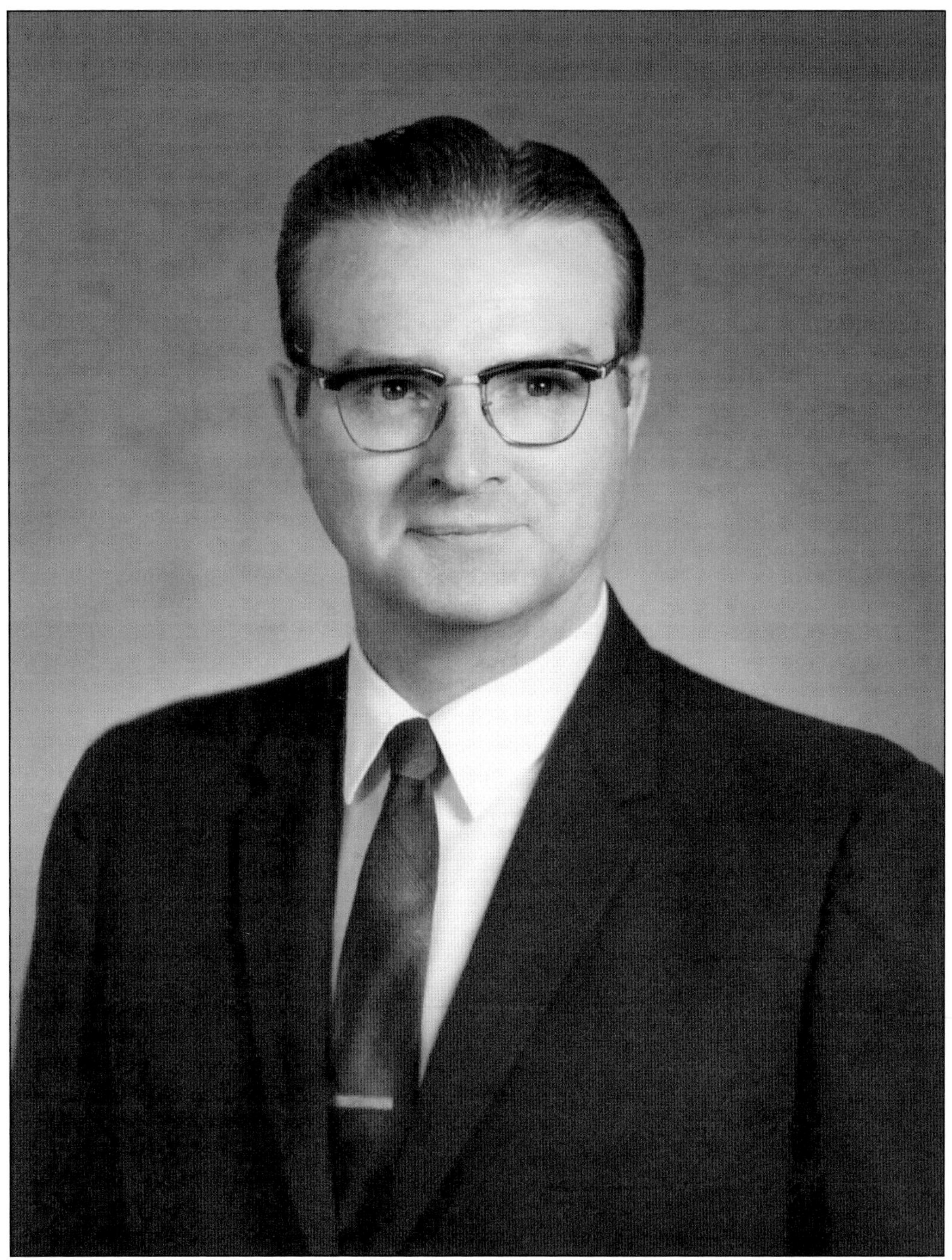

Dr. Laverne Campbell was a Navy veteran of World War II and served as regional health director of the Buffalo office of the New York State Health Department. He also served as medical director and vice president of BlueCross BlueShield of Western New York.

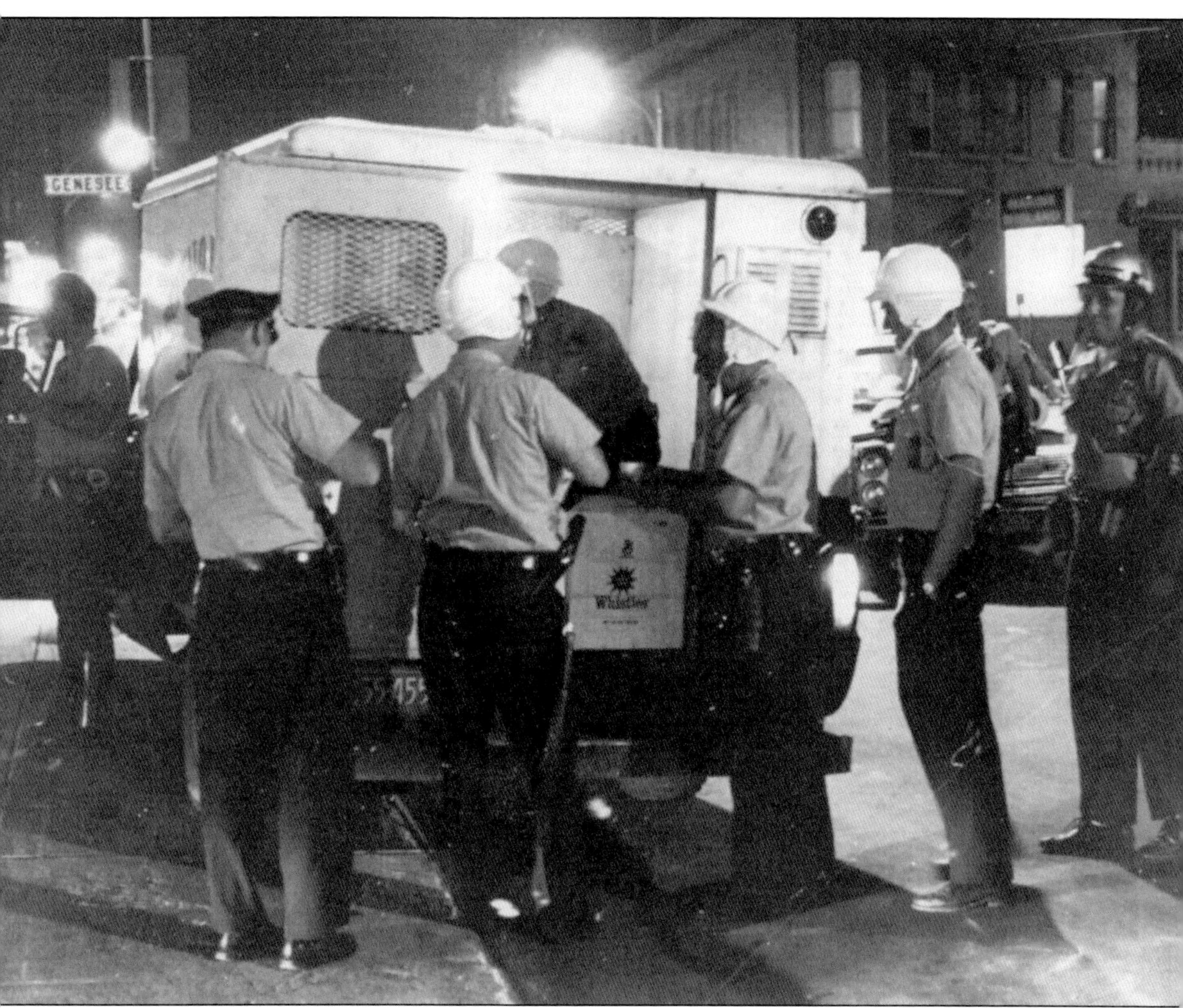

Police are in riot gear near a police van off Genesee Street in Buffalo during the civil rights movement in 1967. According to reports at the time, the Buffalo riot took place on the east side beginning on June 26, and shut down the city. The five-day disturbance resulted in 60 injuries, nearly 200 arrests, and $250,000 in damage. (Courtesy of the Buffalo History Museum, General Photograph Collection, Police–Crimes.)

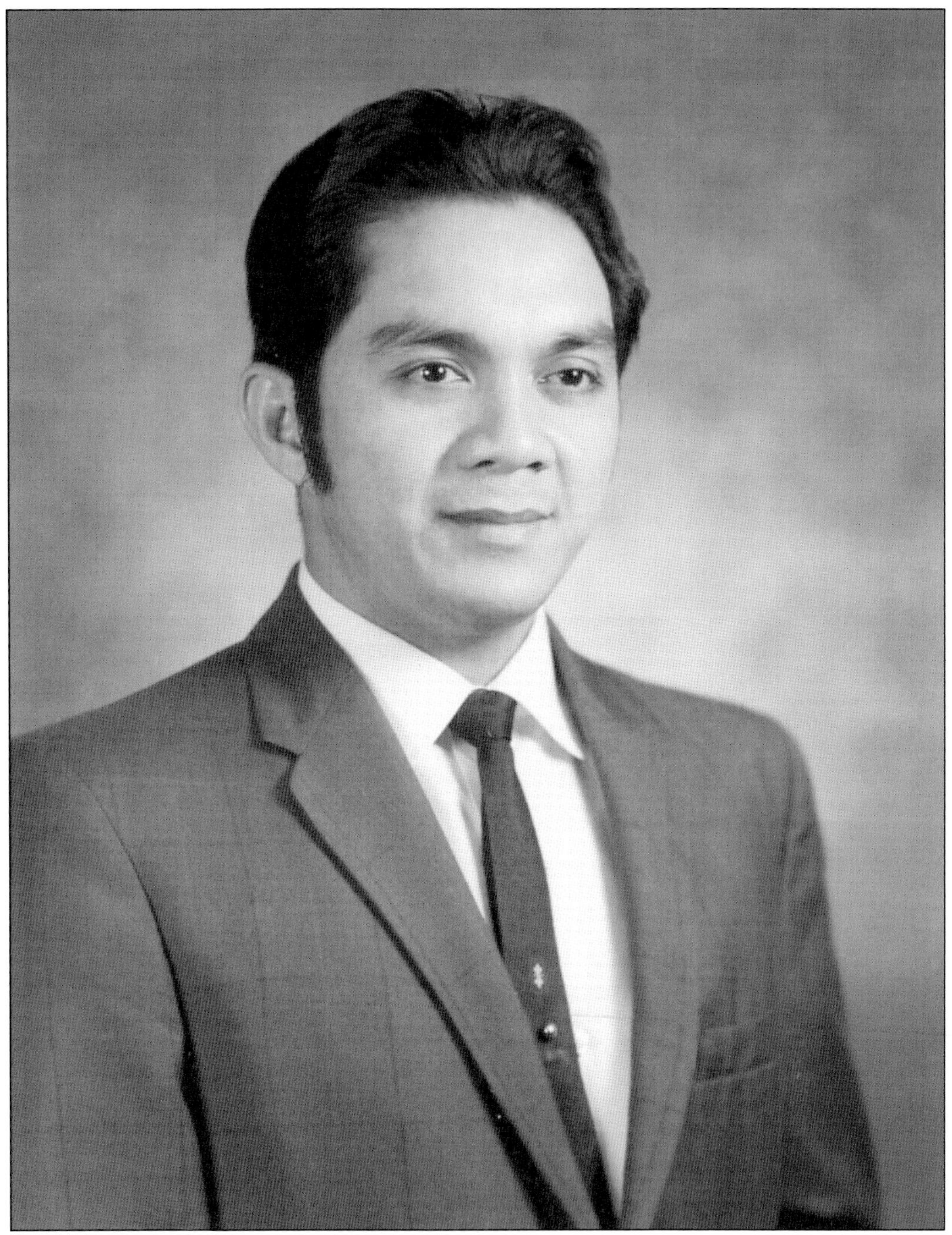

Born in the Philippines, Dr. Eladio Menorca was a Medical Society of Erie County physician-member and served as a urologist where he trained at Millard Fillmore Hospital in New York. He applied for membership at the Medical Society of Erie County on March 13, 1969, and remained a member until his passing on July 6, 2016.

Six

The 1970s

No other natural disaster is linked as closely to Buffalo history as the Blizzard of 1977. The western New York area was hit by a massive snowstorm from January 28 to February 1. Wind gusts ranged from 46 to 69 miles per hour, and the snowfall was recorded as 100 inches in some areas across the region. The high winds blew snow into drifts of 30-40 feet, making travel close to impossible. By the end of the blizzard, Buffalo had lost a total of 29 people in storm-related deaths.

Because the snow accumulated so quickly, plows could not keep up. The city became buried in snowdrifts, and many drivers were stranded in their vehicles. Officials have estimated that one out of every five cars within the city was either parked illegally or abandoned due to the snow. Snowmobiles quickly became the only mode of transportation, transporting patients and medical staff to and from hospitals. Medical care team members stranded at local hospitals were placed in the dire situation of providing care to arriving patients needing urgent care, not being able to transport patients out of the hospital, and not having any care team members able to relieve people of duty due to the storm. A perfect storm to stress an already tense situation.

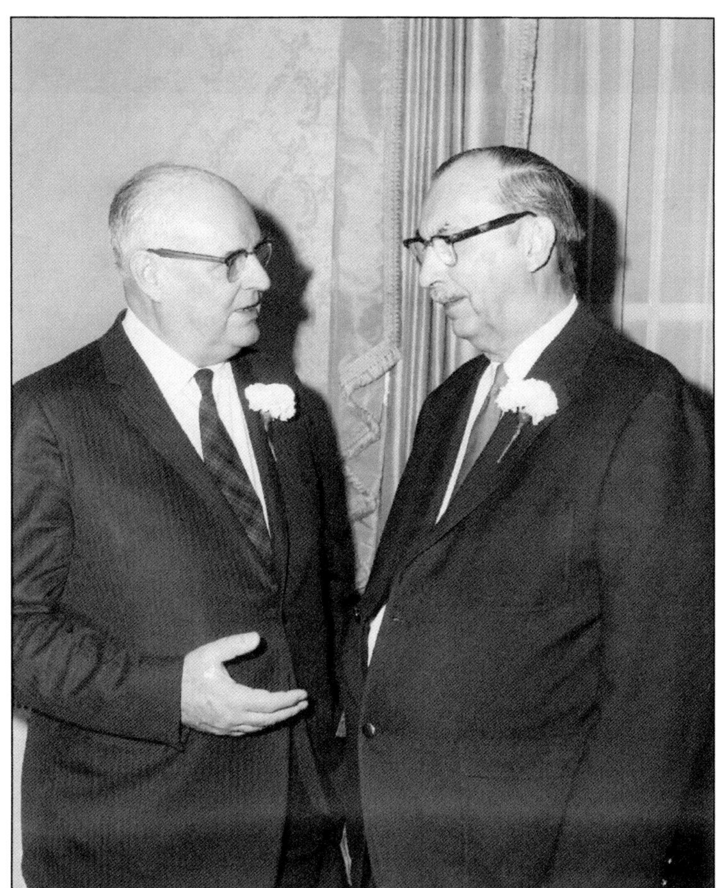

Dr. Walter Walls, Medical Society of Erie County president in 1955, talks with Dr. Carlton Wertz, Medical Society president in 1939. The physicians were attending the Past Presidents' Dinner on May 3, 1970.

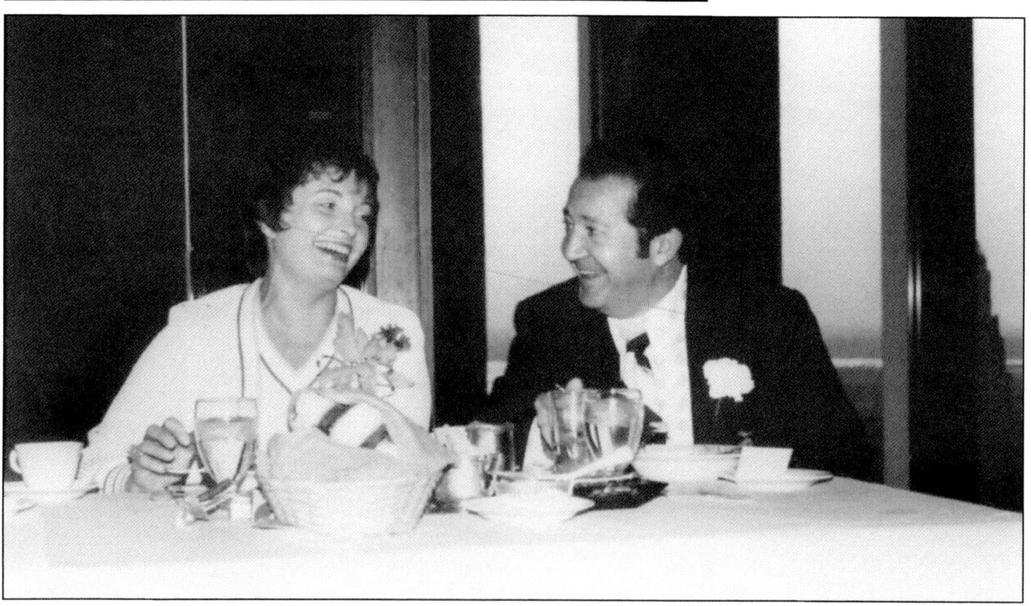

Attending a Medical Society meeting in 1971 are Mrs. Carls, president of the Women's Auxiliary, and Dr. Frank Bolgan, Medical Society president in 1974.

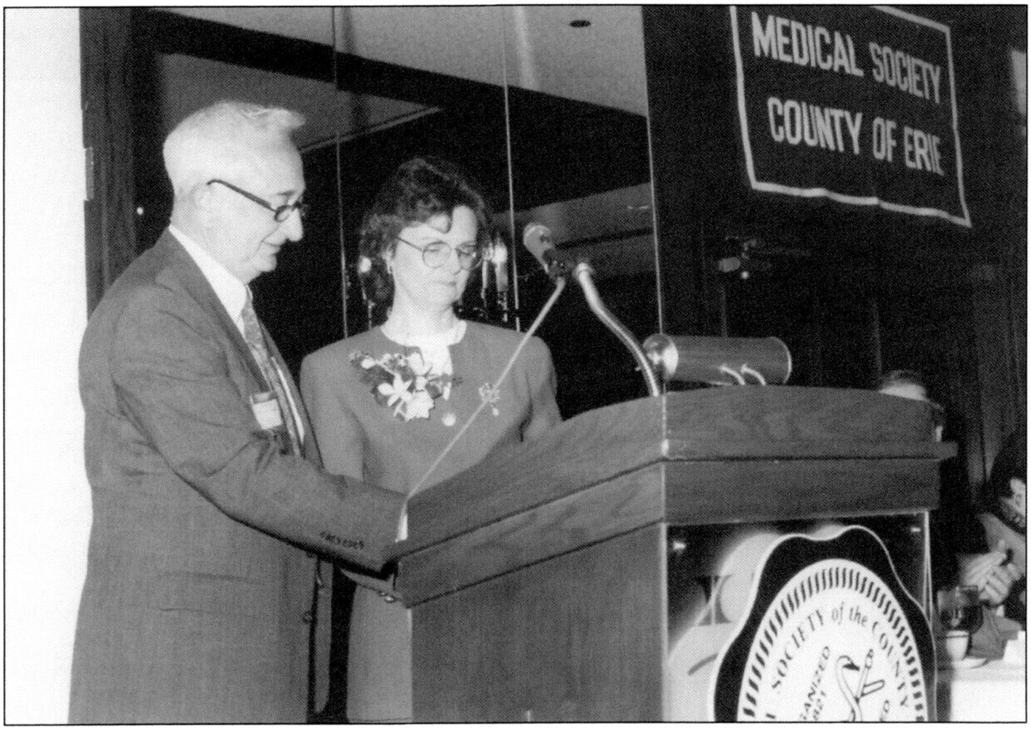

Medical Society president Dr. Anthony Santomauro (1971) is standing at a podium with Dr. Irene Snow, who served as president in 1995. Dr. Snow started her medical career at Buffalo General Medical Center in 1983, joined Buffalo Medical Group in 1988 as a primary care physician, and spent 17 years as medical director. During her tenure, Dr. Snow helped to grow Buffalo Medical Group into a multispecialty practice with more than 200 practitioners.

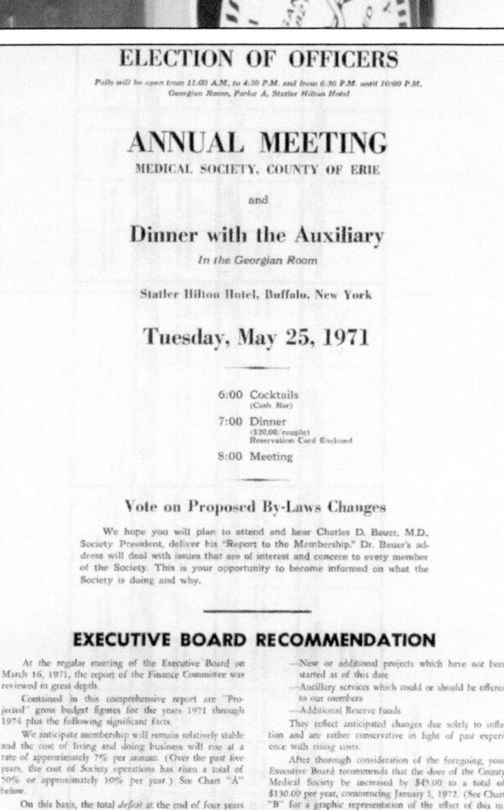

ELECTION OF OFFICERS

Polls will be open from 11:00 A.M. to 4:30 P.M. and from 6:30 P.M. until 10:00 P.M.
Georgian Room, Parlor A, Statler Hilton Hotel

ANNUAL MEETING

MEDICAL SOCIETY, COUNTY OF ERIE

and

Dinner with the Auxiliary

In the Georgian Room

Statler Hilton Hotel, Buffalo, New York

Tuesday, May 25, 1971

6:00 Cocktails
(Cash Bar)

7:00 Dinner
($20.00/couple)
Reservation Card Enclosed

8:00 Meeting

Vote on Proposed By-Laws Changes

We hope you will plan to attend and hear Charles D. Bauer, M.D., Society President, deliver his "Report to the Membership." Dr. Bauer's address will deal with issues that are of interest and concern to every member of the Society. This is your opportunity to become informed on what the Society is doing and why.

EXECUTIVE BOARD RECOMMENDATION

At the regular meeting of the Executive Board on March 16, 1971, the report of the Finance Committee was reviewed in great depth.

Contained in this comprehensive report are "Projected" gross budget figures for the years 1971 through 1974 plus the following significant facts.

We anticipate membership will remain relatively stable and the cost of living and doing business will rise at a rate of approximately 7% per annum. (Over the past five years, the cost of Society operations has risen a total of 30% or approximately 10% per year.) See Chart "A" below.

On this basis, the total *deficit* at the end of four years would be *$104,628.00*.

The figures projected in the report do not include any of the following —

—New or additional projects which have not been started as of this date

—Ancillary services which could or should be offered to our members

—Additional Reserve funds

They reflect anticipated changes due solely to inflation and are rather conservative in light of past experience with rising costs.

After thorough consideration of the foregoing, your Executive Board recommends that the dues of the County Medical Society be increased by $45.00 to a total of $130.00 per year, commencing January 1, 1972. (See Chart "B" for a graphic representation of the effect of this increase.)

A comparison of MSCE dues to other dues across the state is depicted in Chart "C".

This is an annual meeting notice marking the 150th anniversary of the Medical Society in 1971. The event consisted of a cocktail hour and dinner followed by a meeting where members would vote on proposed bylaw changes. The notification also advised members of an executive board recommendation that membership dues be increased to $130 per year. Today, dues are $815 per year.

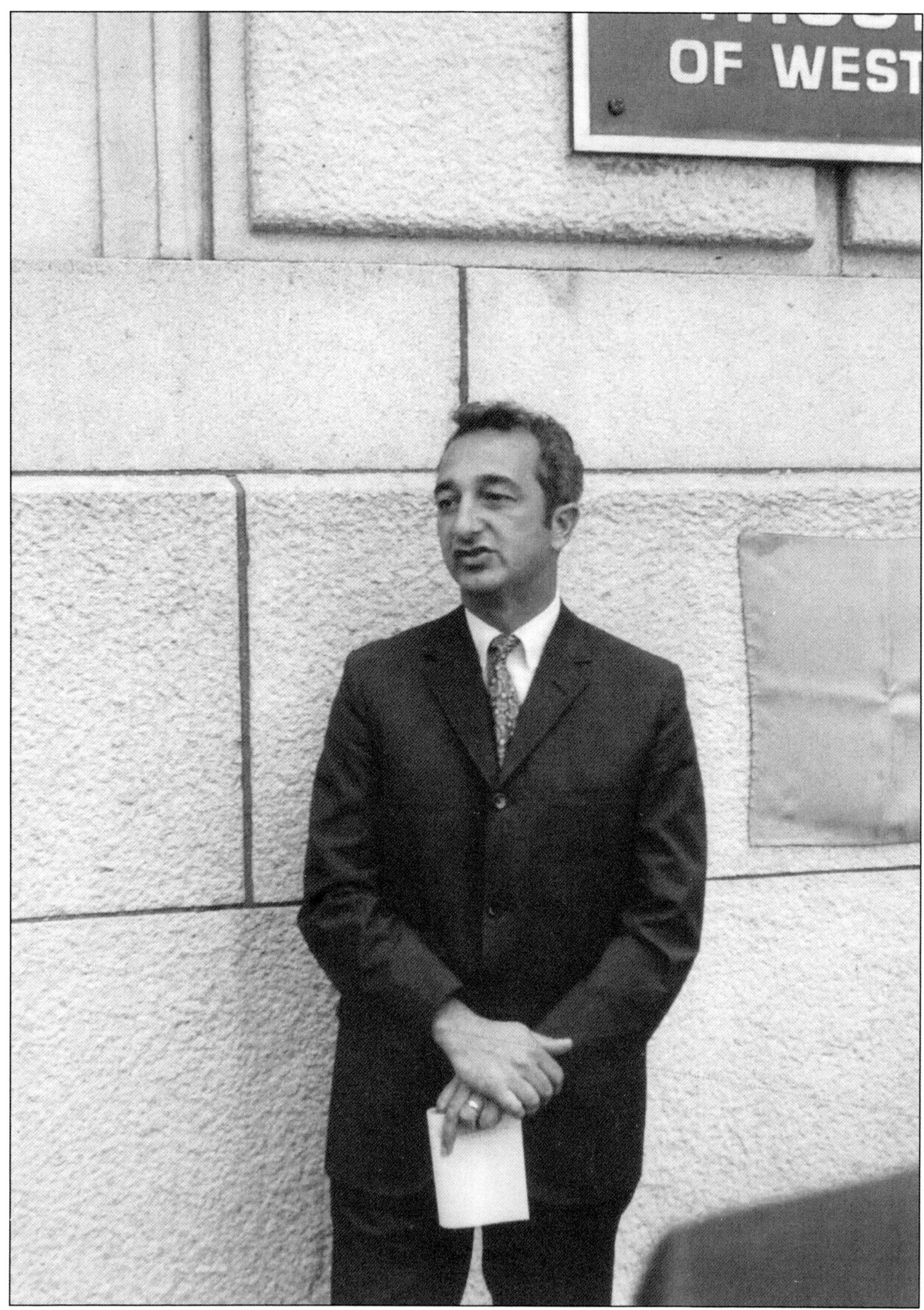

Pictured here is the unveiling of the Medical Society of Erie County plaque at its original home at 237 Main Street in Buffalo. There to unveil the plaque was Dr. Anthony Santomauro, president of the Medical Society from 1971 to 1972. The plaque remains today.

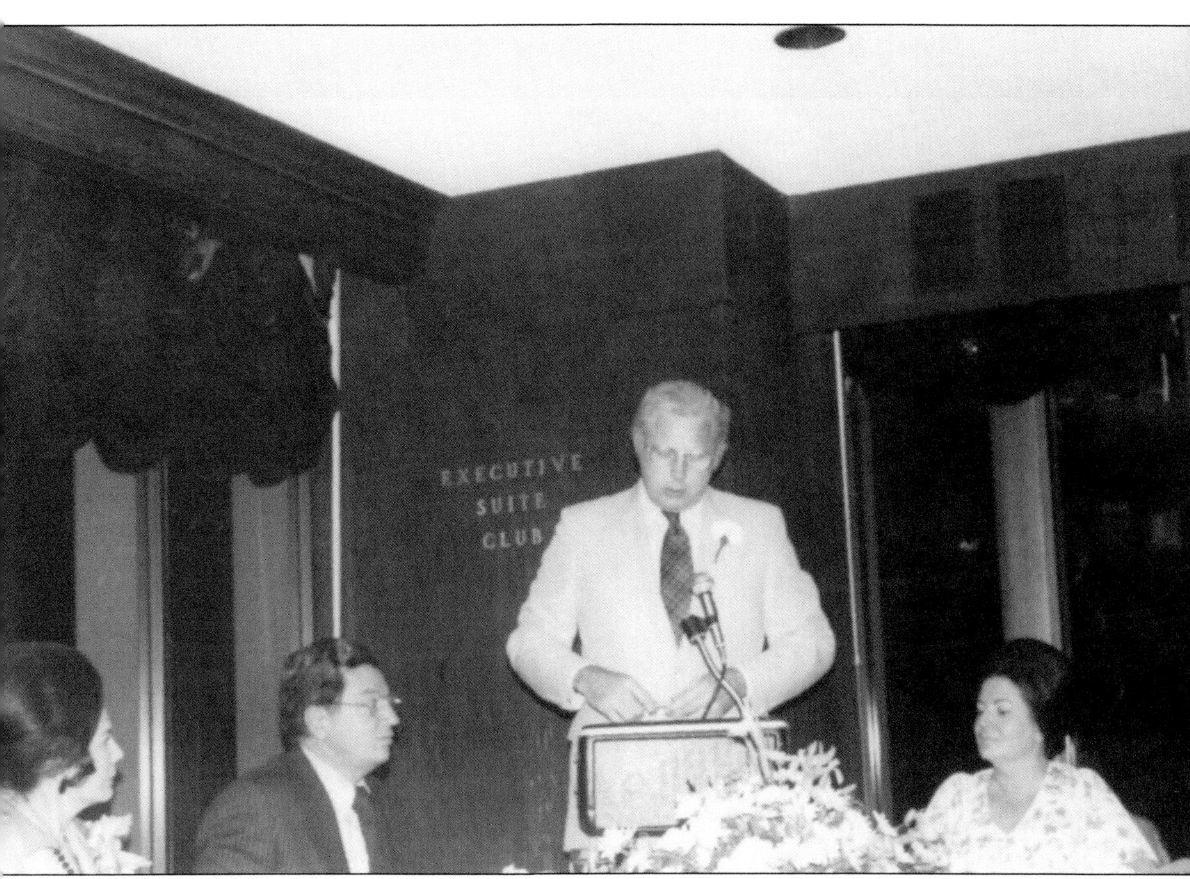

Dr. James Cosgriff Jr. is presenting at the annual meeting of the Medical Society of Erie County. He was president from 1973 to 1974. Dr. Cosgriff also held offices in the American College of Surgeons on both the state and local levels, the American College of Emergency Physicians, and the Buffalo Surgical Society.

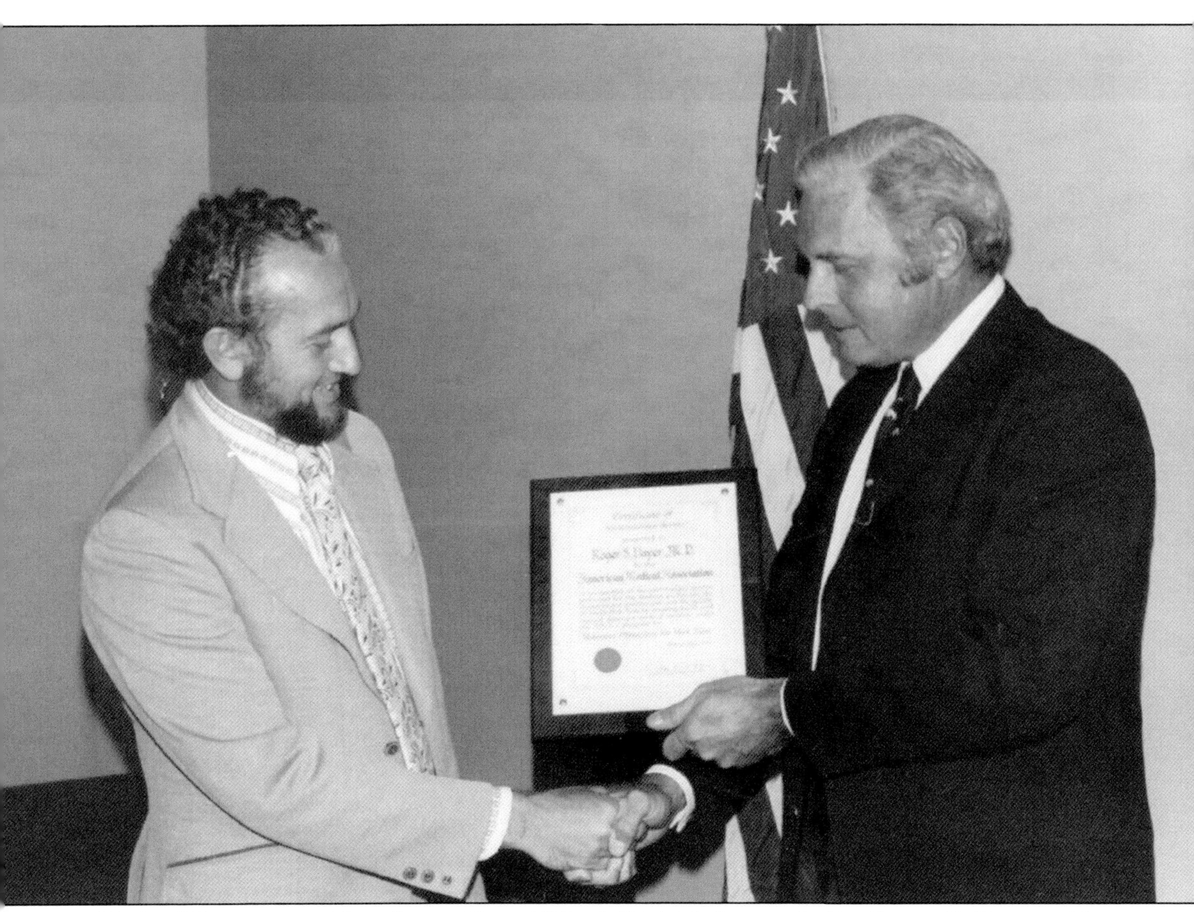

Medical Society president James Cosgriff Jr., MD (right), awards Dr. Roger S. Dayer with a Certificate of Humanitarian Service issued by the American Medical Association for Dayer's volunteer service to treat the ill in Vietnam. Dr. Cosgriff was vice chairman of the Council on Ethical and Judicial Affairs of the American Medical Association.

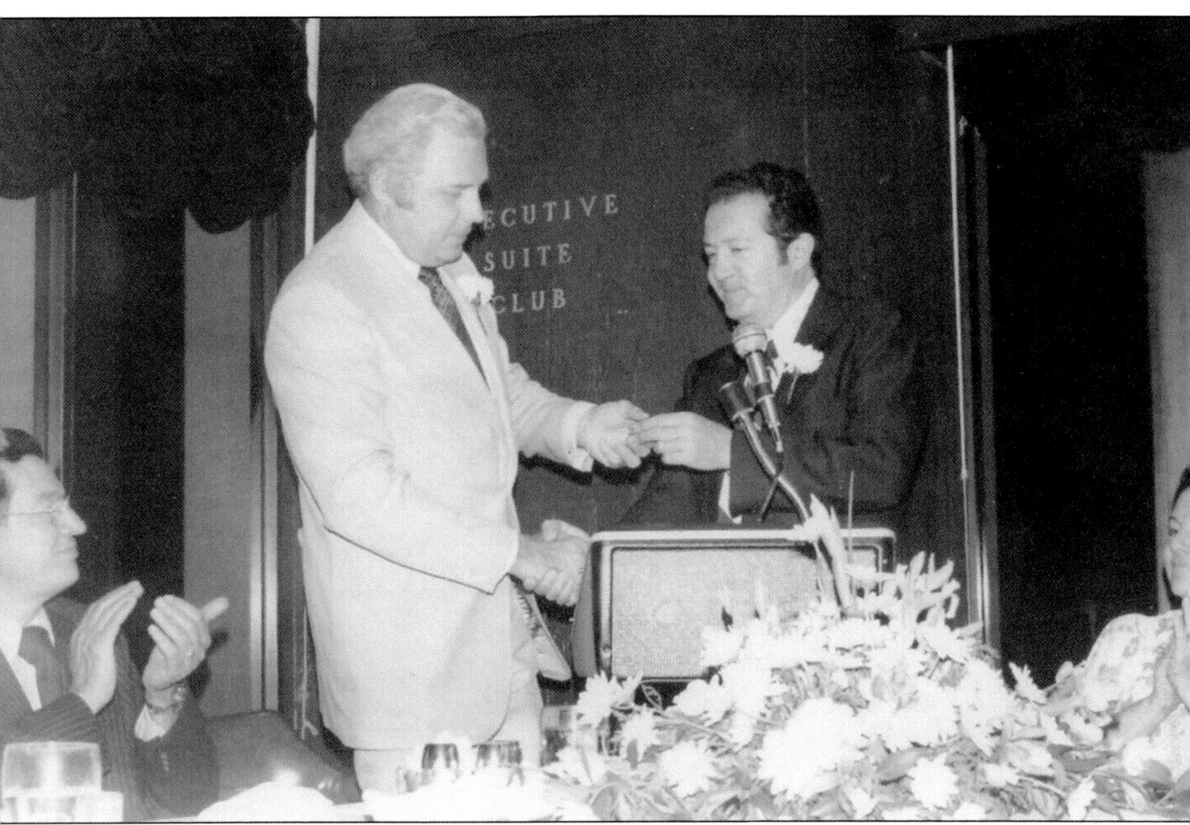

Dr. James Cosgriff Jr. was an internationally renowned Buffalo surgeon and president of the Medical Society of the State of New York from 1994 to 1995. Dr. Cosgriff published more than 100 papers and presentations at local, national, and international medical meetings and conferences. He served in the Navy from 1944 to 1946, was a graduate of Canisius College in 1947, and a 1951 cum laude graduate of the Georgetown School of Medicine. He was chief resident of surgery at E.J. Meyer Memorial Hospital, now the Erie County Medical Center.

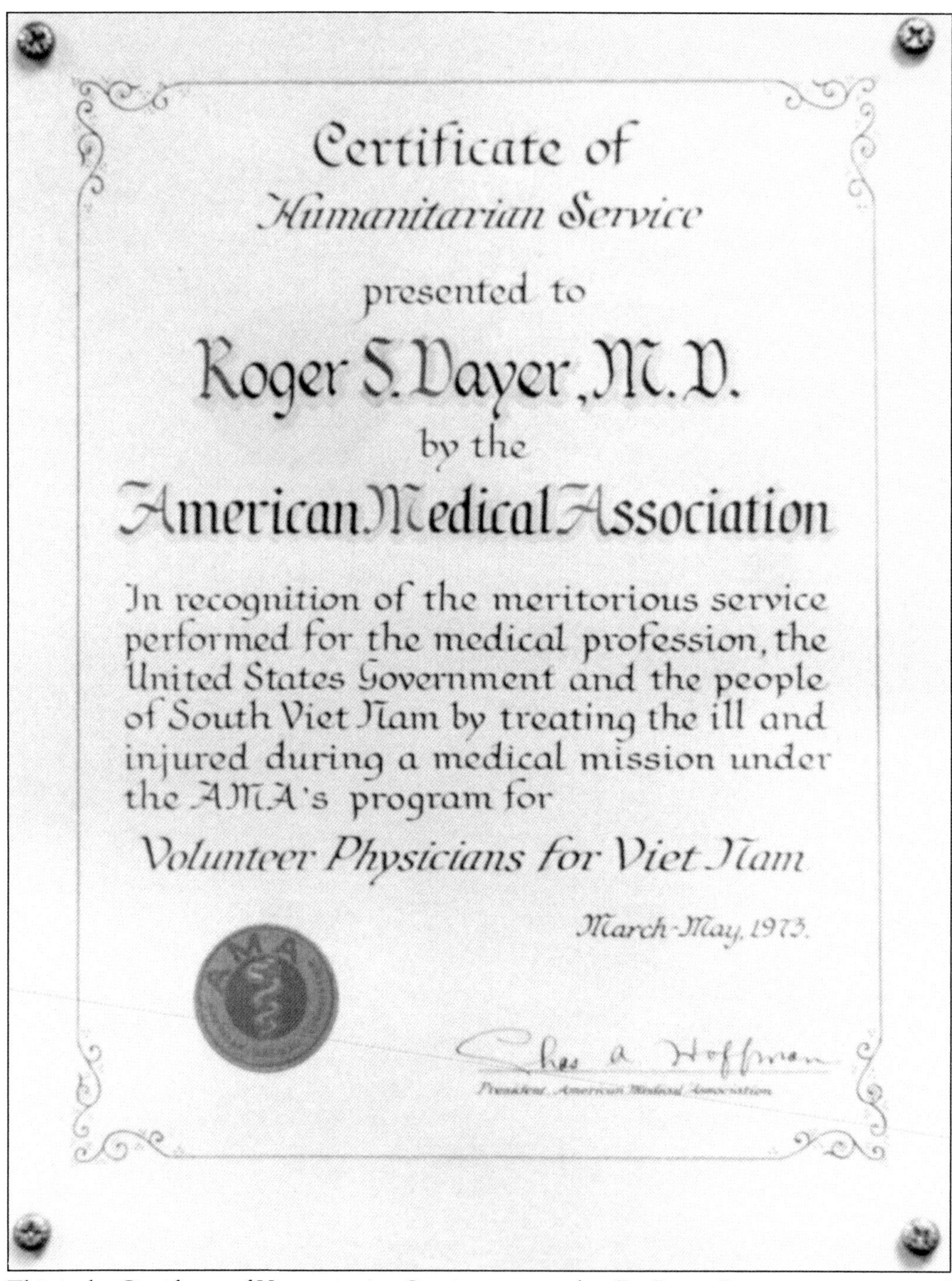

Certificate of
Humanitarian Service
presented to
Roger S. Dayer, M.D.
by the
American Medical Association

In recognition of the meritorious service performed for the medical profession, the United States Government and the people of South Viet Nam by treating the ill and injured during a medical mission under the AMA's program for

Volunteer Physicians for Viet Nam

March-May, 1973.

President, American Medical Association

This is the Certificate of Humanitarian Service presented to Dr. Roger Dayer in recognition of his commendable volunteer medical service in South Vietnam. Dr. Dayer served as part of the Volunteer Physicians for Viet Nam from March to May 1973.

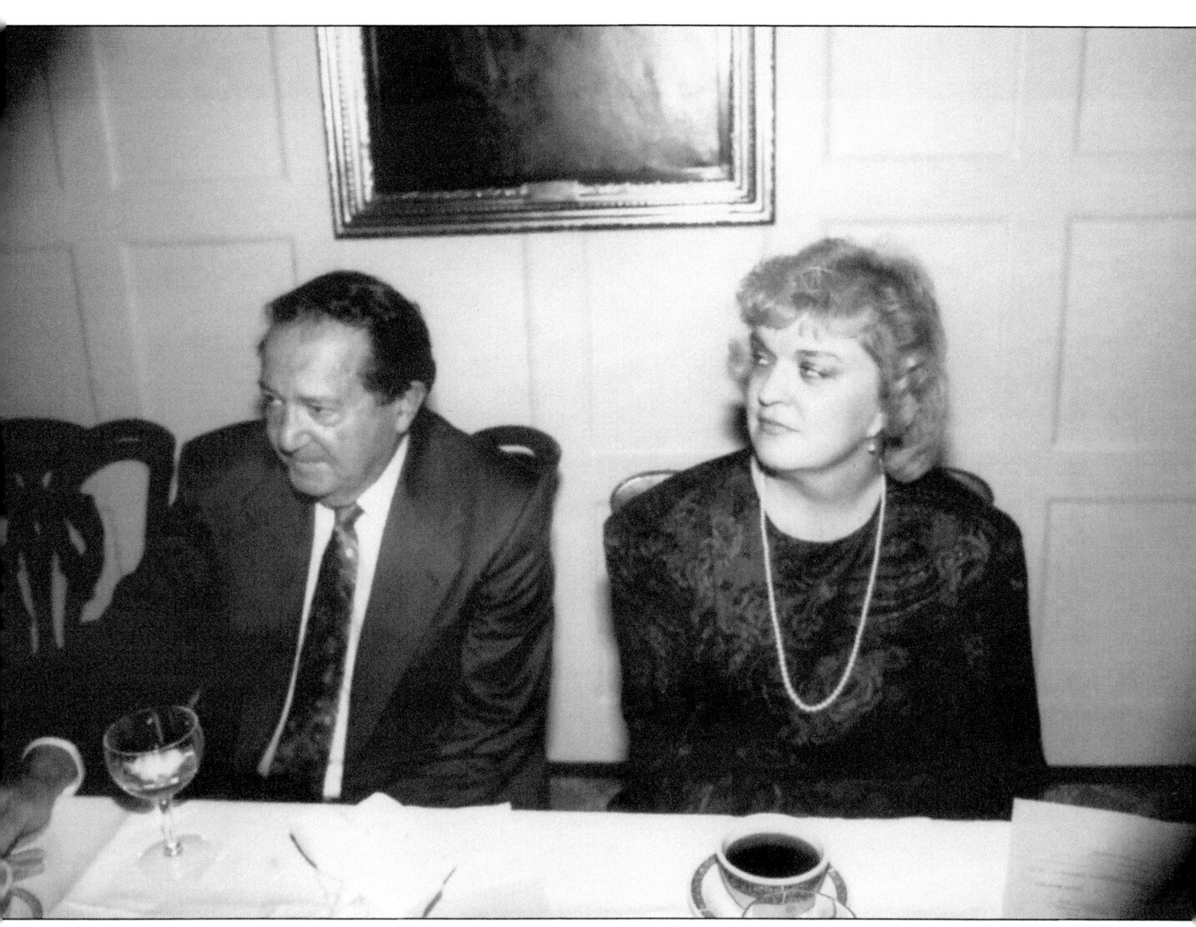

Shown with Dr. Frank Bolgan, Medical Society president in 1974, is Dr. Nancy Nielson, the first female president of the Medical Society in 1989, at an annual meeting dinner. Dr. Nielson also served with distinction as the first female speaker of the House of Delegates of the Medical Society of the State of New York and of the American Medical Association. Dr. Nielson, a female physician pioneer, was the second female president of the American Medical Association.

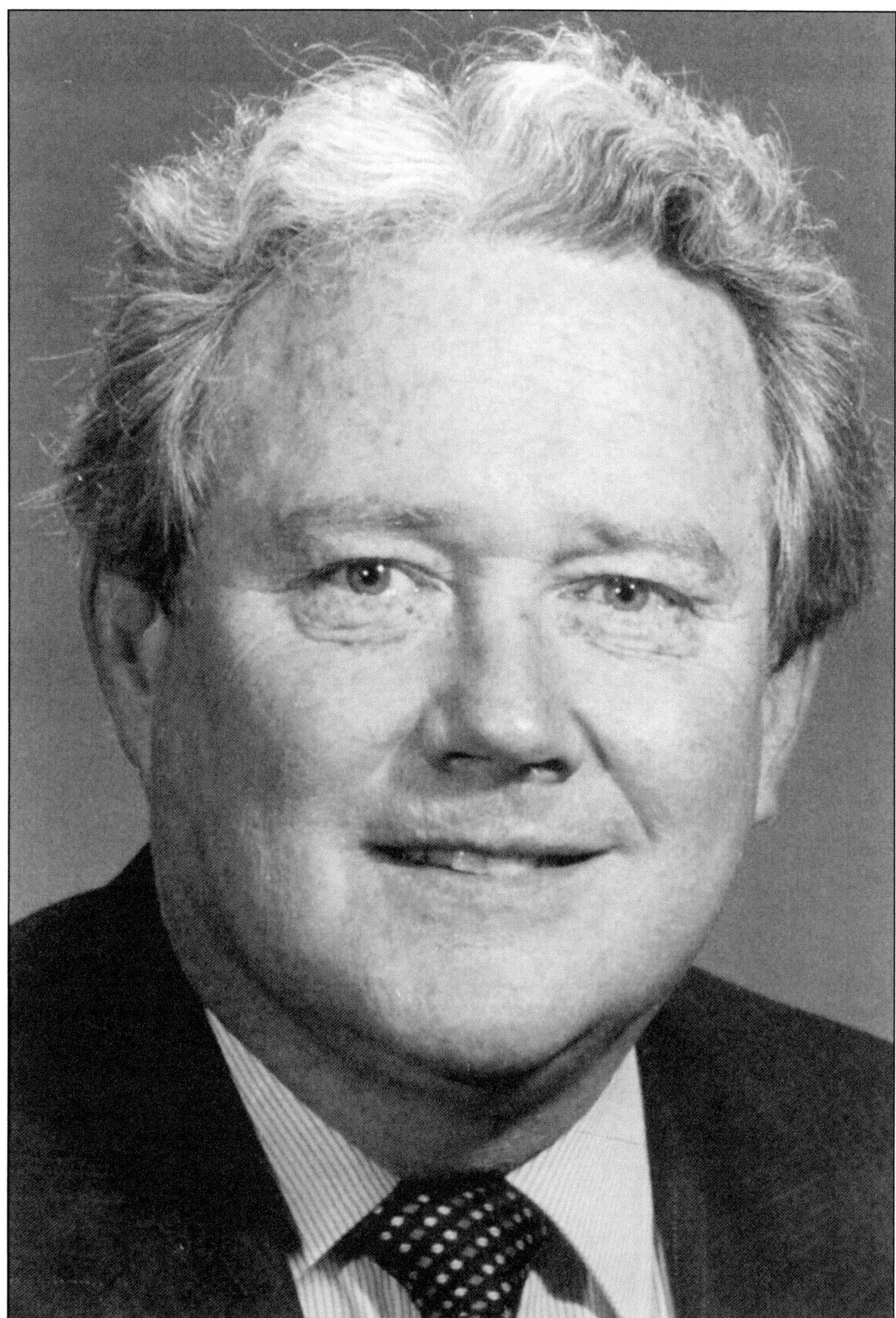

Dr. John Naughton was the longest serving dean in the history of the School of Medicine and Biomedical Sciences (1975–1996), as it is known now. He was one of the key players in establishing the University at Buffalo's innovative consortium of teaching hospitals, a model that subsequently garnered national attention as a new approach to medical education. (Courtesy of University Archives, University at Buffalo.)

Seven

Our Journey Continues

Erie County has continued to evolve, and in 2001, a major development took place with the rise of the Buffalo Niagara Medical Campus, which has been a means to foster collaboration between the medical organizations within the region and a platform for continued urban growth, community outreach, medical innovation, and excellence in care for the citizens of the county.

The evolution of Erie County has been expansive, starting from a small town of only a few settlers to a national leader in innovation and excellence. The story of this region does not stop here, though. It continues to grow and develop as the journey to this point in time has taken us through both triumphs and tragedies. The Medical Society of Erie County continues to stand ready, willing, and able to serve, meeting whatever challenges tomorrow will bring.

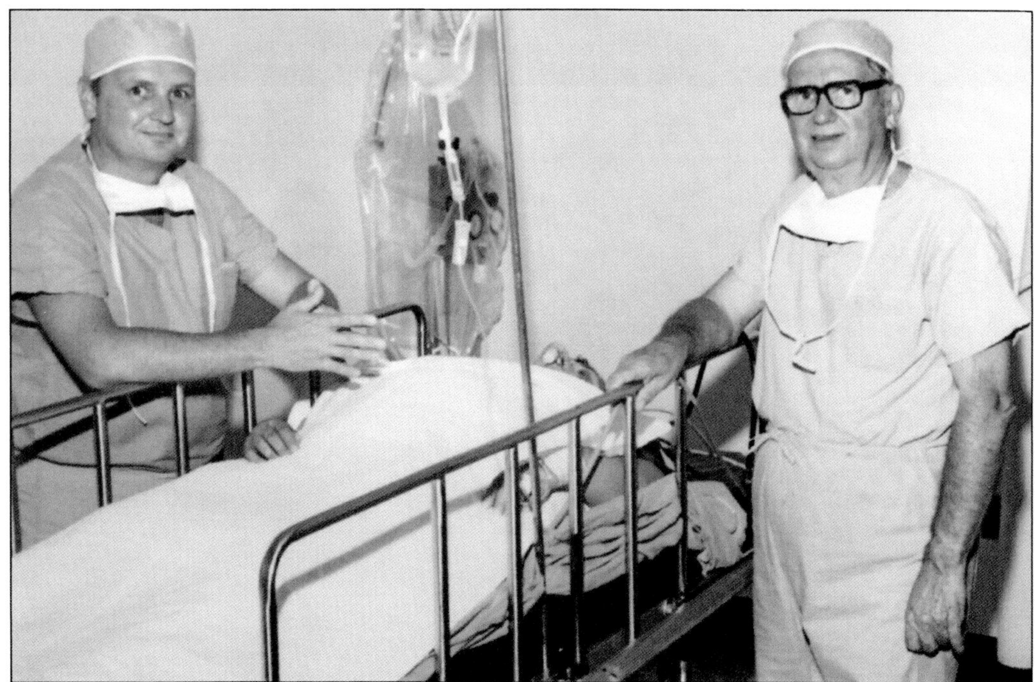

Kenneth Eckhert Jr., MD (left), Medical Society president in 2004–2005, stands with his father, Dr. Kenneth Eckhert (right), president in 1960–1961, while working together at Deaconess Hospital in the 1980s. The elder Dr. Eckhert is the grandfather to Medical Society president Kenneth Eckhert III, MD (2019), and was a well-renowned physician-leader throughout the region.

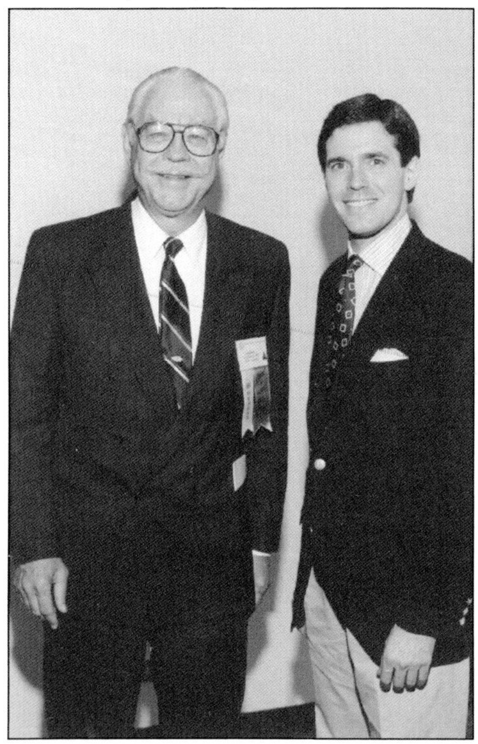

Medical Society member Dr. Edmund J. Gicewicz (left) was a standout football, basketball, and baseball player for the University of Buffalo and was elected to the University of Buffalo Athletics Hall of Fame in 1966 and the Greater Buffalo Sports Hall of Fame in 1999. He served as the football team physician for nearly three decades and was president of the University at Buffalo Medical Alumni Association, the founder and first medical director of the University Sports Medicine Institute, and an assistant professor of clinical surgery and orthopedics at Jacobs School of Medicine. Dr. Gicewicz was honored with the Distinguished Alumni Award in 1977, the prestigious Samuel Capen Chancellor's Award in 1978, and the University at Buffalo President's Medal in 2013.

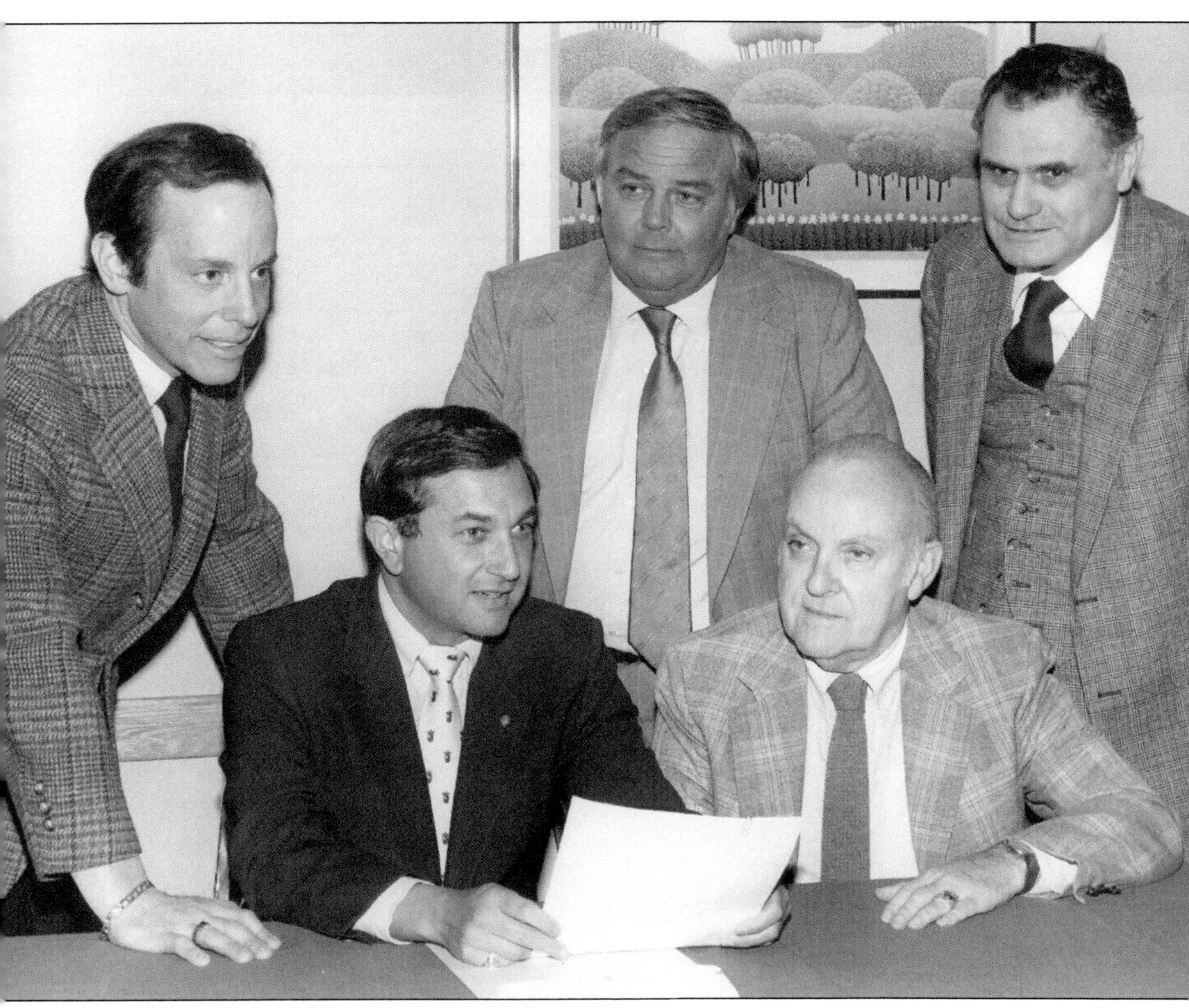

From left to right are David Davidson of the Podiatry Society of New York, Dr. Robert Chick of the Eighth District Dental Society, William Dowd of the Eighth District Dental Society, Dr. Leo Manning (Medical Society president in 1985), and James Coppola of the Pharmacists Association of Western New York. These men came together at a forum created by the Medical Society of Erie County to discuss mutual problems affecting their professions.

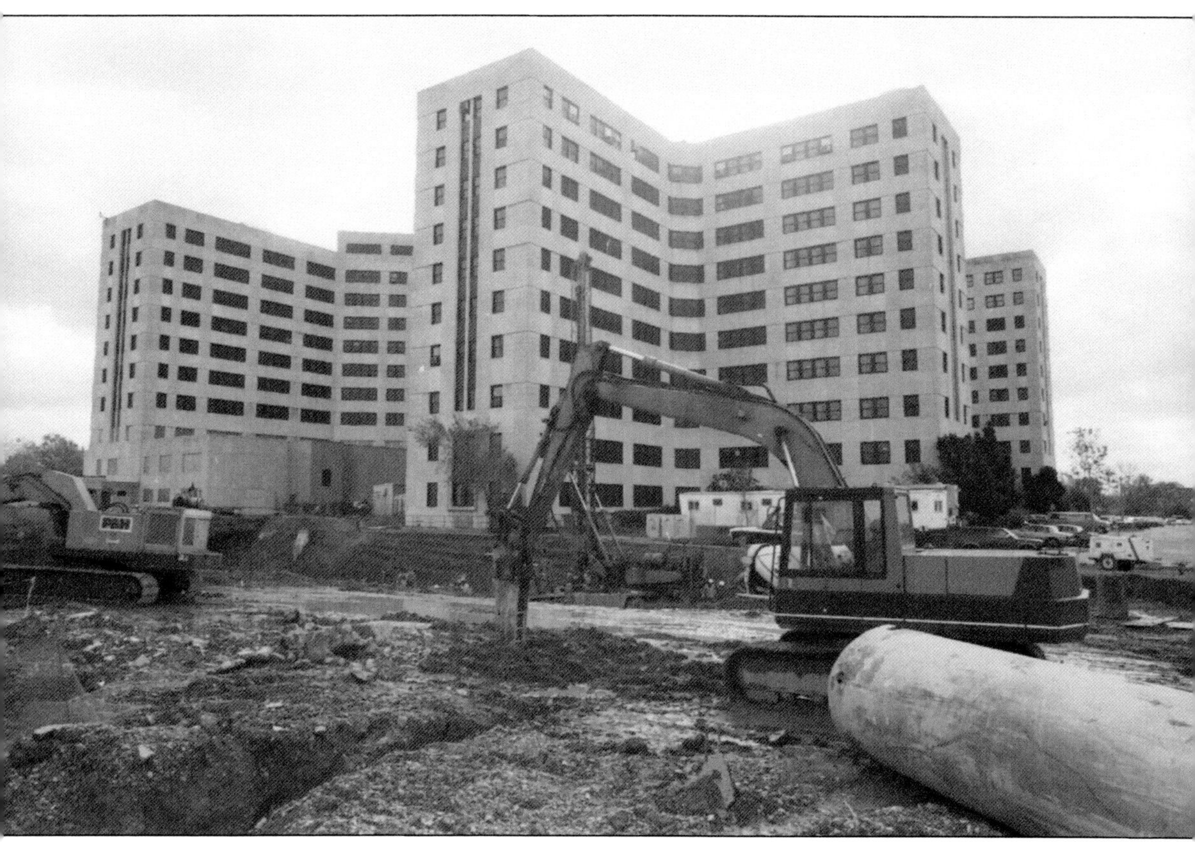

Pictured here is the VA Hospital undergoing construction in 1988. Medical Society president Dr. Abraham Aaron, 1945, prioritized the best possible care for veterans. On October 18, 1945, President Truman approved a 1,000-bed hospital for Buffalo, and Grover Cleveland Park was chosen as the site. Buffalo's VA Hospital was the first 1,000-bed structure in the United States to be opened under the VA's postwar building program and treated some 6,000 patients in the first year after it opened. (Courtesy of University Archives, University at Buffalo.)

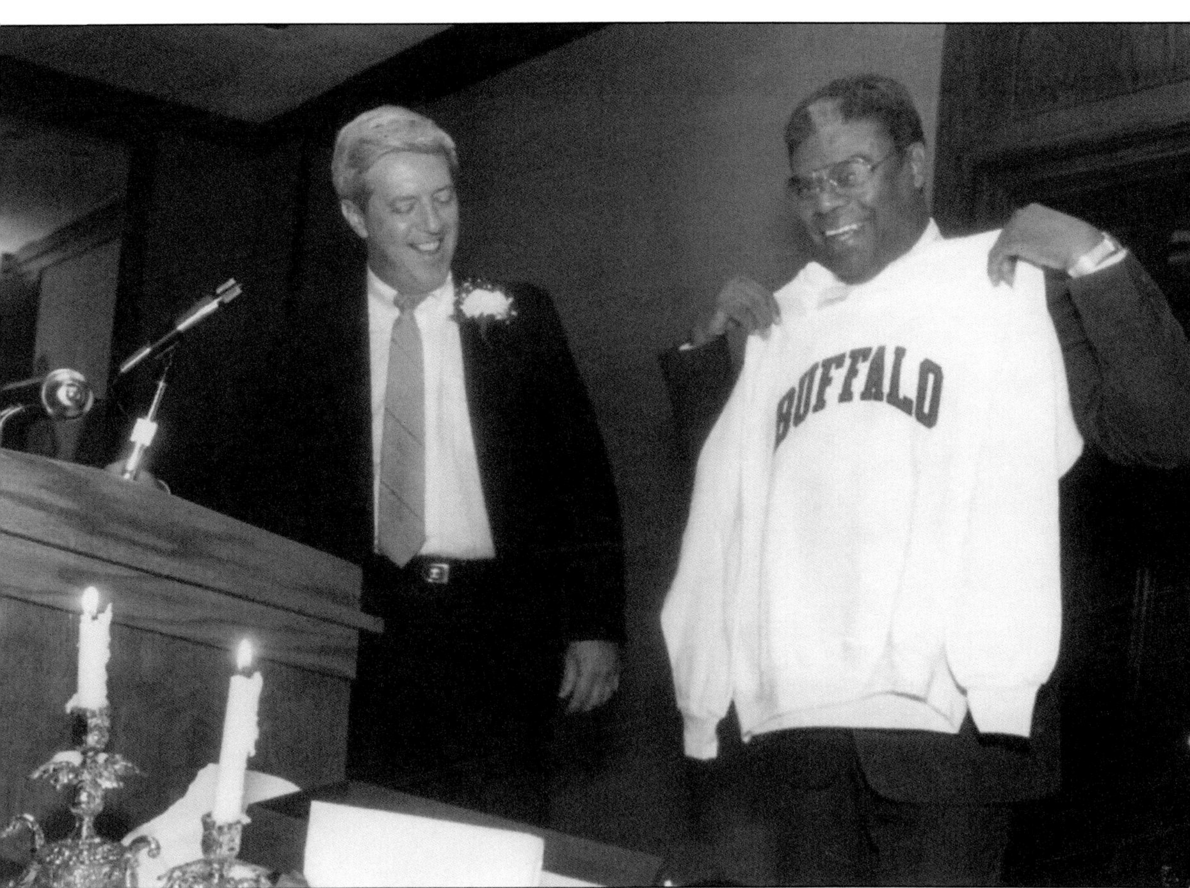

Seen here with 1991 Medical Society president William "Skip" Major (left) is Percy Wootton, a cardiologist who became president of the American Medical Association in 1997. Dr. Wootton graduated from the Medical College of Virginia in 1957 and was a fellow of the American College of Physicians and the American College of Cardiology.

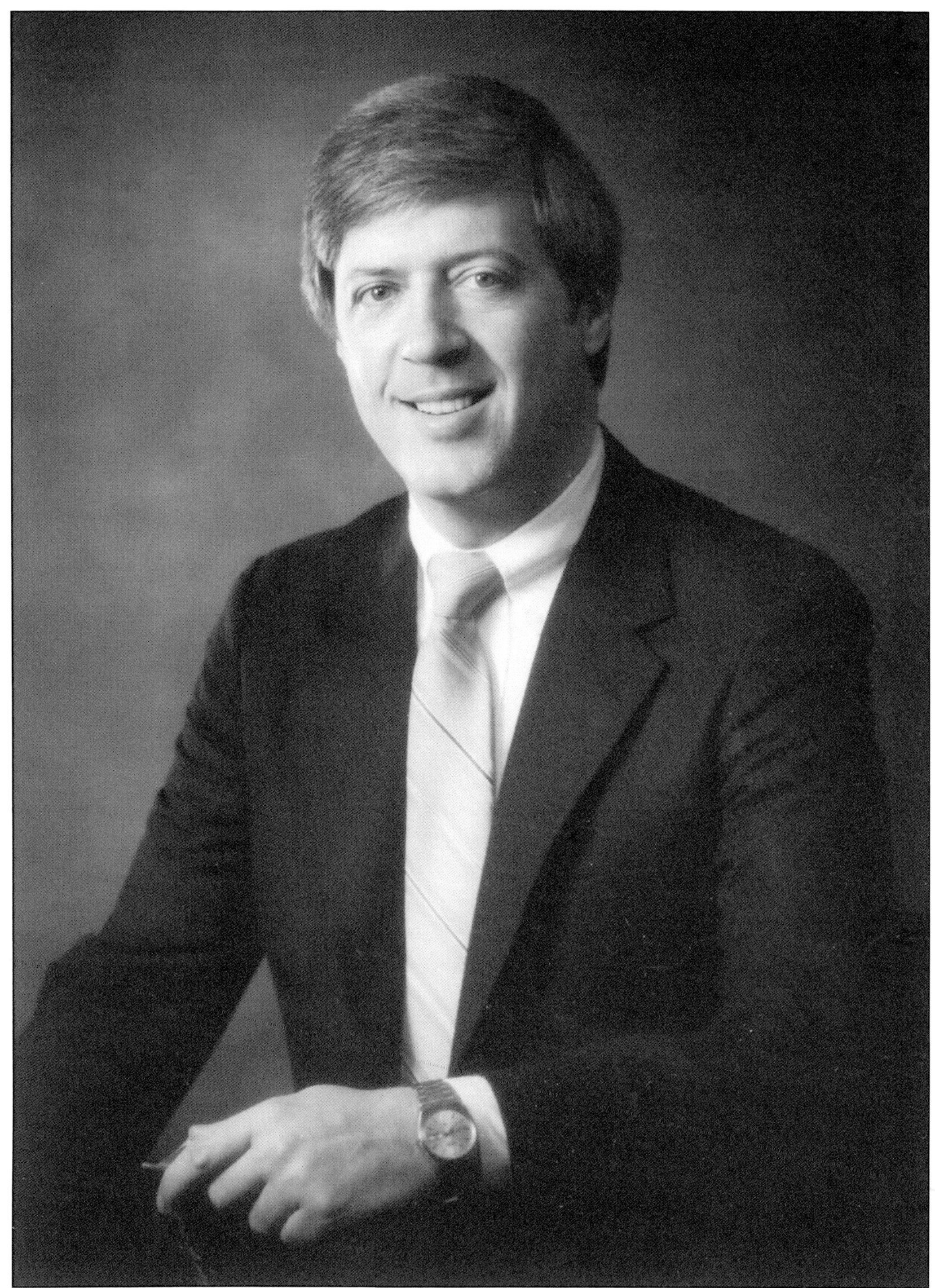

Dr. William "Skip" Major was a prominent surgeon and health care executive in Buffalo. He was active in physician advocacy issues and served as president of the Medical Society in 1989. He was appointed to the Board for Professional Medical Conduct in 1991 and was awarded the James H. Cosgriff Jr. Distinguished Leadership Award by the Medical Society.

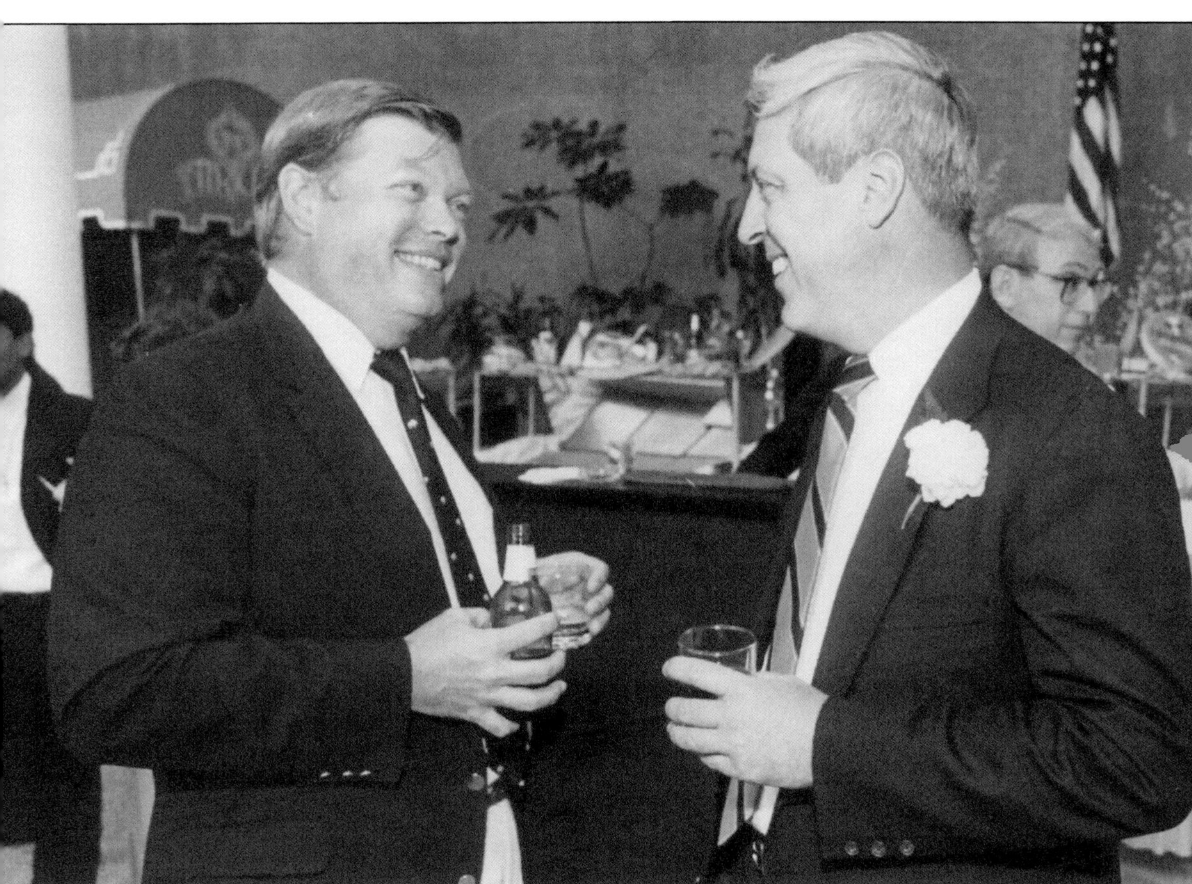

Pictured here are Dr. William "Skip" Major (right) with fellow member Dr. Evan Evans at a Medical Society function. Dr. Major served as medical director of Independent Health. From 1999 to 2005, he was the executive director of IPA/WNY, a physician organization that provides medical services to independent health subscribers. Dr. Evans was a general surgeon who was well regarded for minimally invasive surgical techniques on the abdomen.

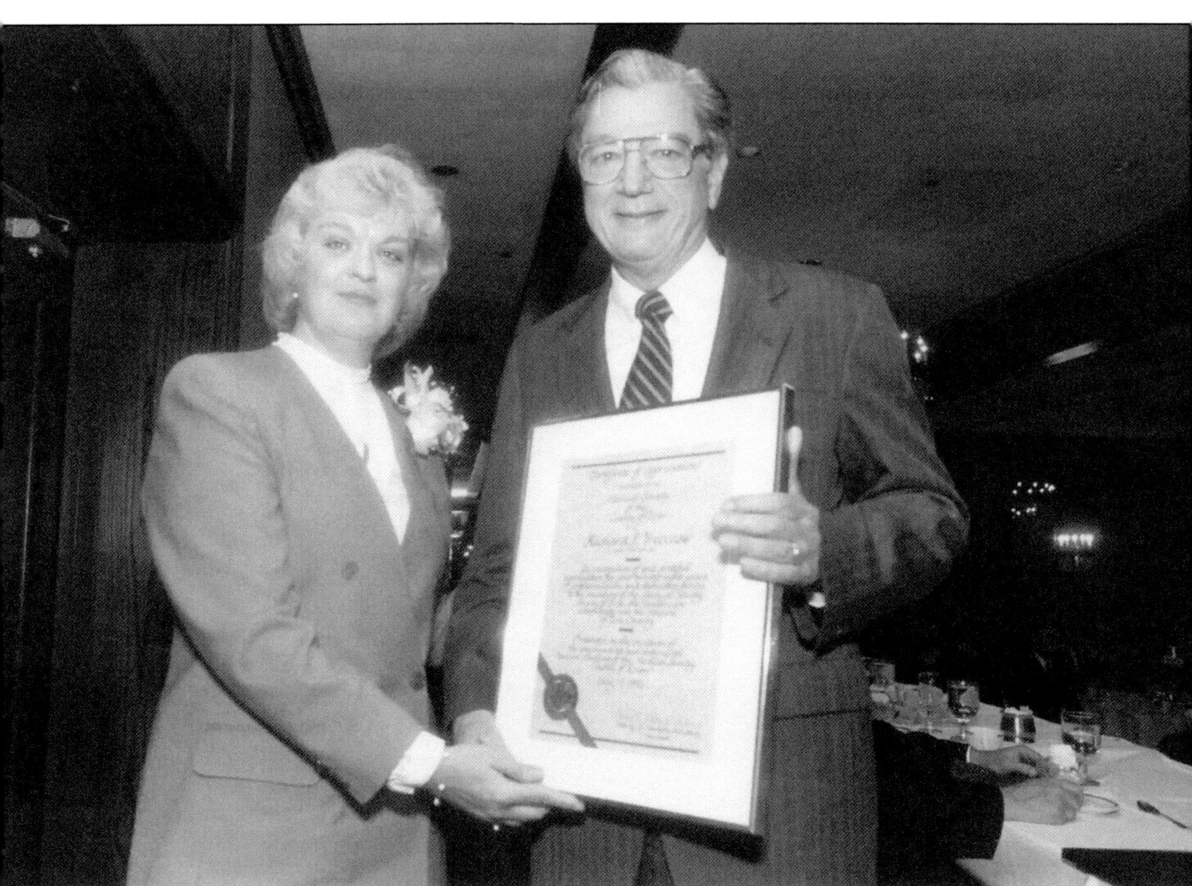

Pictured here is Nancy Nielsen, MD, PHD, the first female president of the Medical Society of Erie County and the second female president of the American Medical Association. Dr. Nielsen is awarding Richard Trecasse, executive director of the Medical Society, a certificate of appreciation for his years of service.

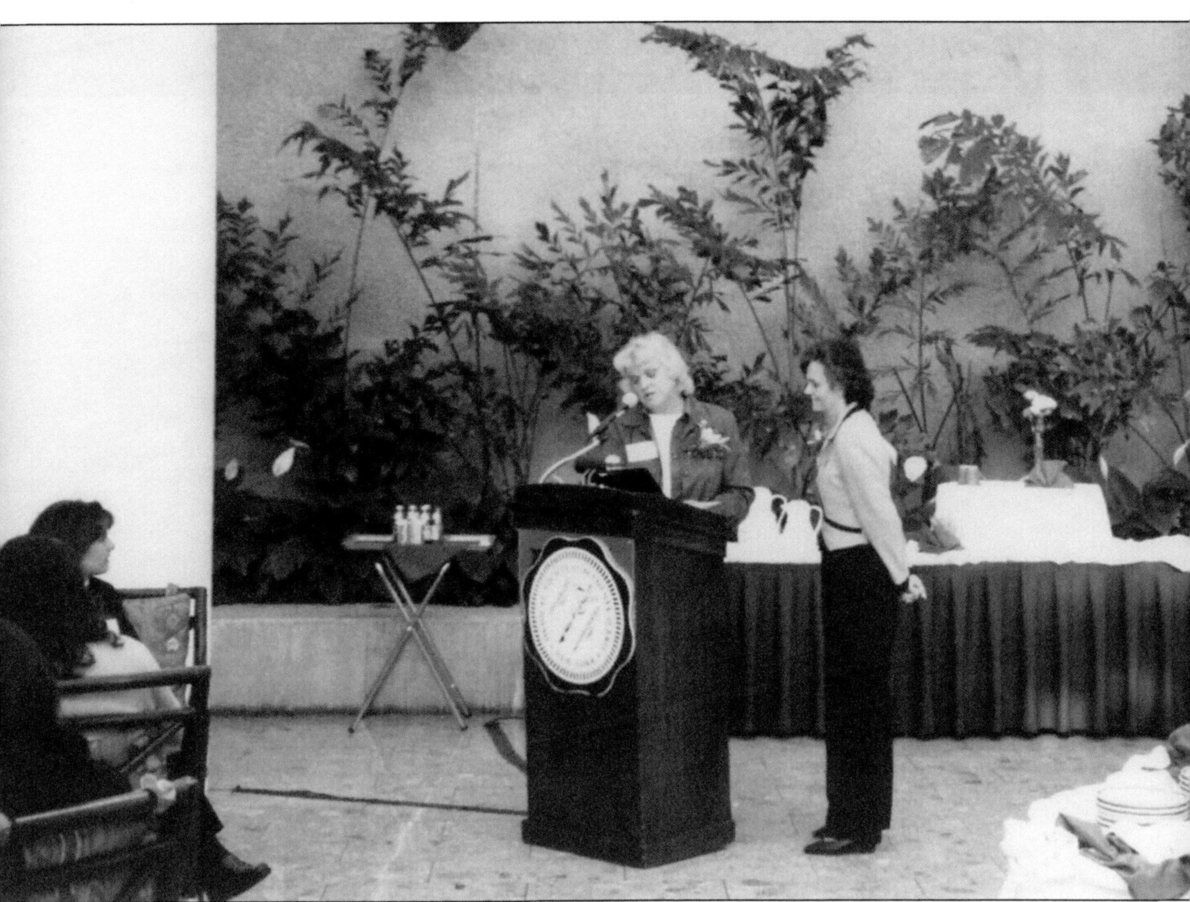

Pictured here are Dr. Nancy Nielsen (left) with Dr. Irene Snow, president of the Medical Society of Erie County (1995–1996), at an annual meeting event. Dr. Nielsen served as senior advisor to the Center for Medicare and Medicaid Innovation, sat on the National Institutes of Health Advisory Committee on Research on Women's Health from 2008 to 2011, served as World Medical Association delegate from the American Medical Association until 2010, cochaired Racial/Ethnic Disparities Advisory Board until 2009, served as invited faculty to George Washington University School of Public Health from 2013 to 2017, and was an invited lecturer at New York University Robert F. Wagner Graduate School of Public Service. Her honors and awards include the 2009 Elizabeth Blackwell Award issued by the American Medical Women's Association, induction into West Virginia University's Hall of Fame in 2009, Distinguished Alumnus Award from University at Buffalo School of Medicine in 2008, and numerous lifetime achievement awards.

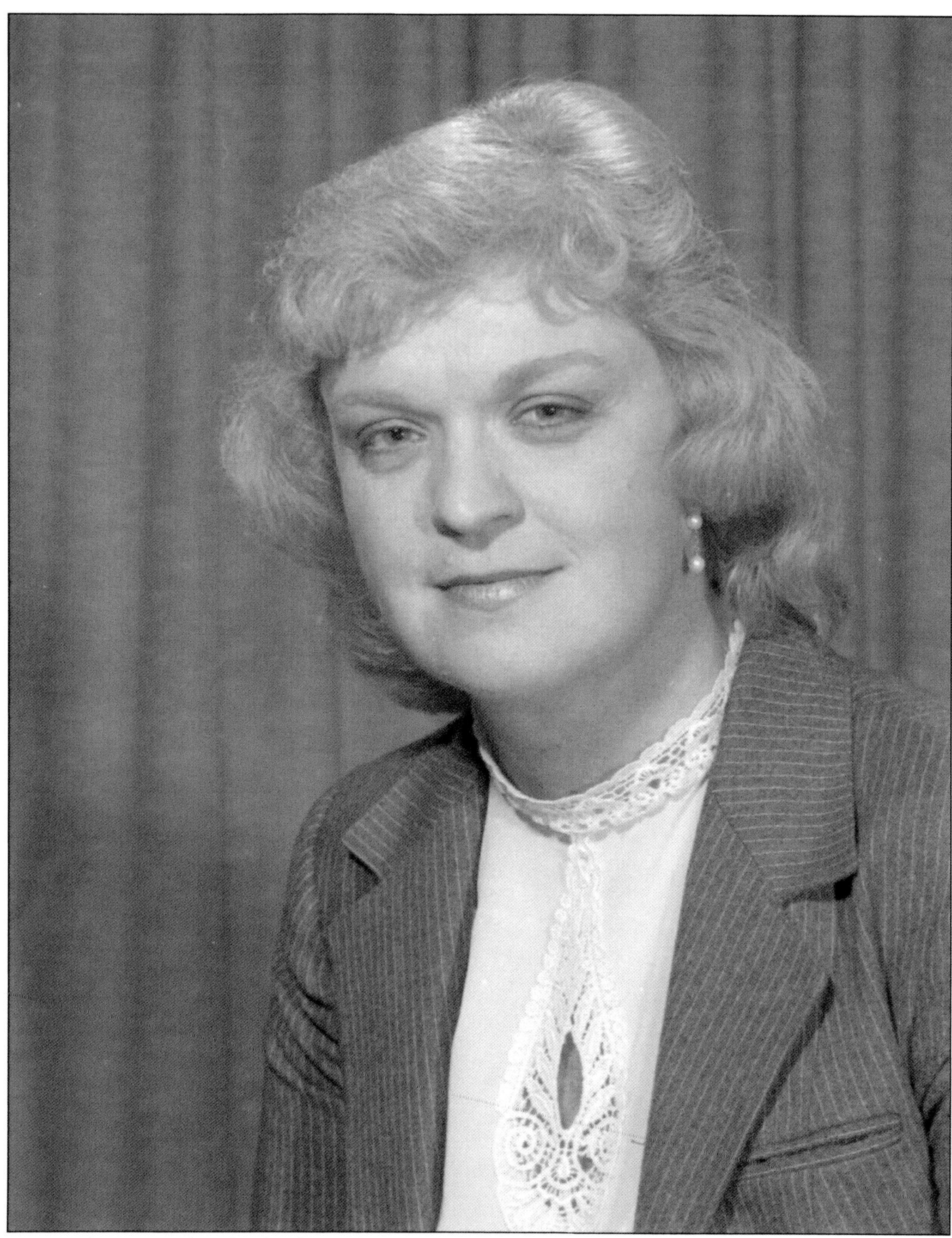

Among her countless leadership roles, Dr. Nielsen served as senior adviser for the Center for Medicare and Medicaid Innovation at the US Department of Health and Human Services (2011–2013), as a board member of FAIR Health Inc., as an elected member to the Institute of Medicine of the National Academies of Science, cochair to the Commission to End Healthcare Disparities, and cochair to the Racial/Ethnic Disparities Advisory Board.

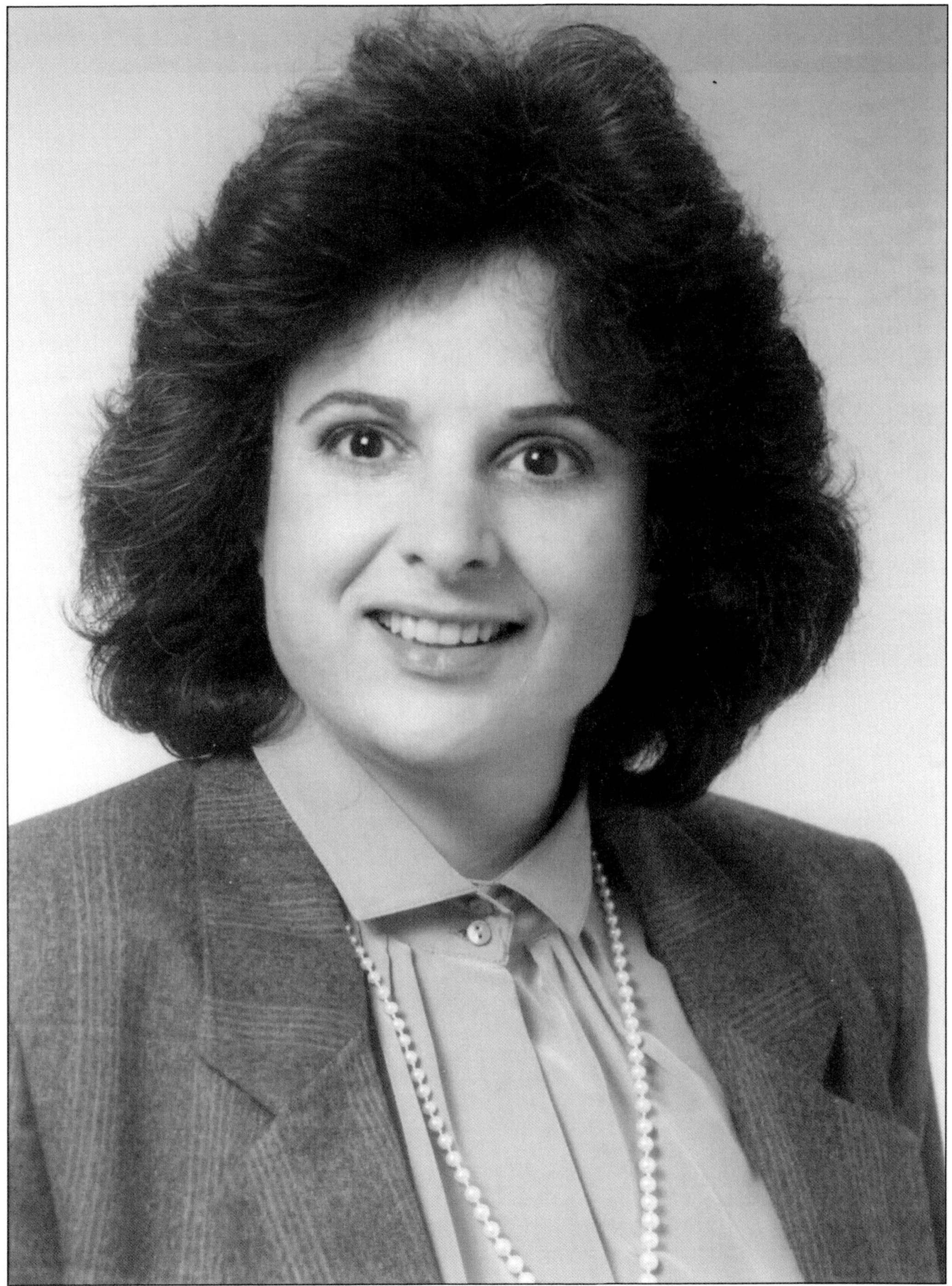

Dr. Amy Early, an oncologist at Roswell Park Comprehensive Cancer Center since 1980, was president of the Medical Society of Erie County in 1991–1992. One of only a few female presidents of the Medical Society in the last 200 years, Dr. Early served as associate professor of oncology at the Jacobs School of Medicine and continues practicing oncology at Roswell Park today. (Courtesy of Gordon Fitzgerald, Gordon James Image Maker.)

Community Service Award
Upstate New York
Transplant Services, Inc.
In recognition of your advancement
of organ and tissue donation and
transplantation within our community.
While fulfilling this mission you
enhance the quality of life for many
residents in need of these most precious gifts.
During 10 years of operation UNYTS
has helped bridge the gap between
the shortage of organ and tissue donors
and the many people awaiting transplant.
Throughout this process you provide
valuable assistance and support to
physicians, nurses, hospital administration,
health associations and the public.
The physician members of the
Medical Society of the County of Erie
commend your achievements
and support your valuable service
to our community.
Medical Society
Presented on

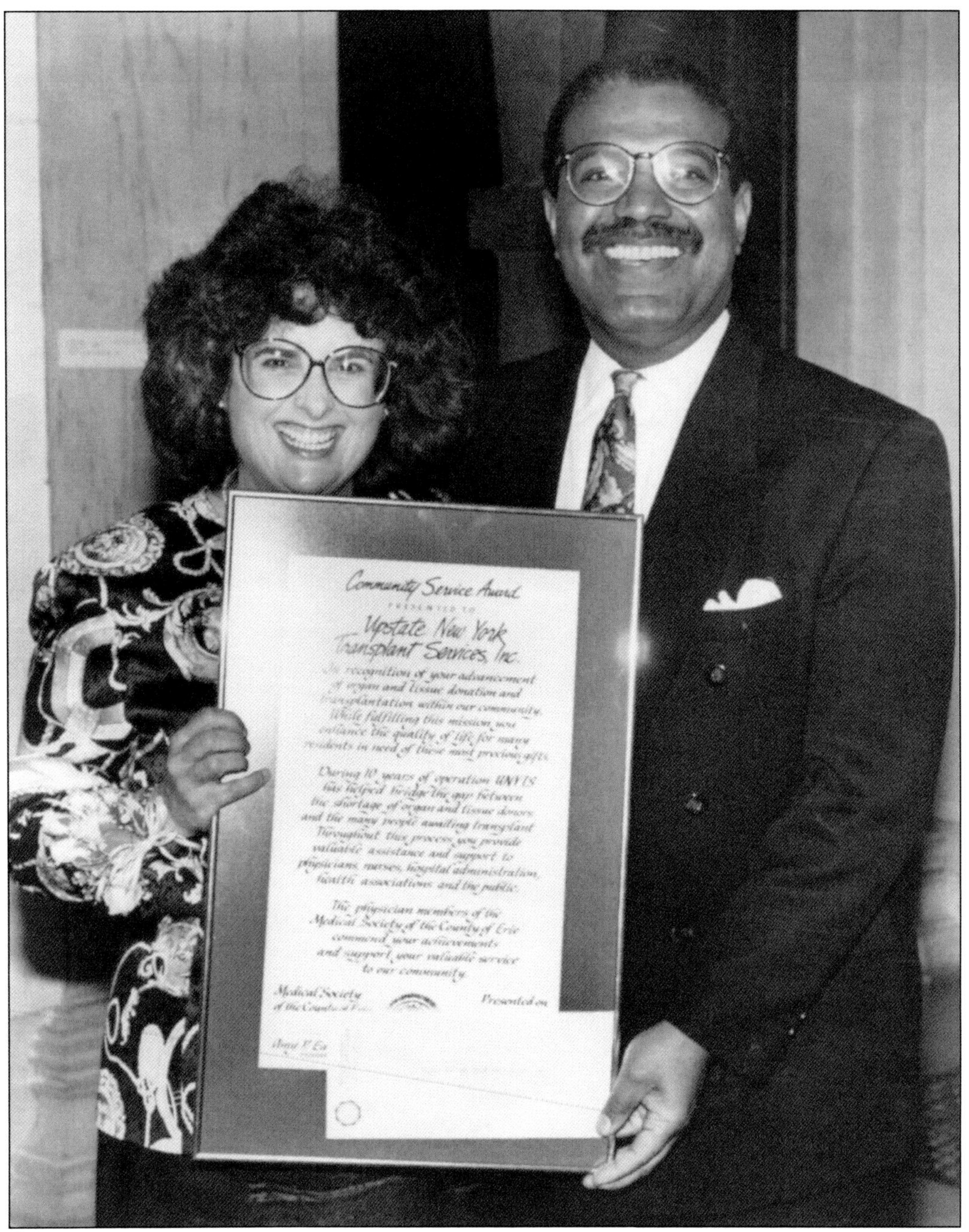

Dr. Amy Early, Medical Society president, presents a representative of the Upstate New York Transplant Service with the Medical Society's Community Service Award in 1991. The Upstate New York Transplant Service is now known as Connect Life Blood and Organ Donor Network.

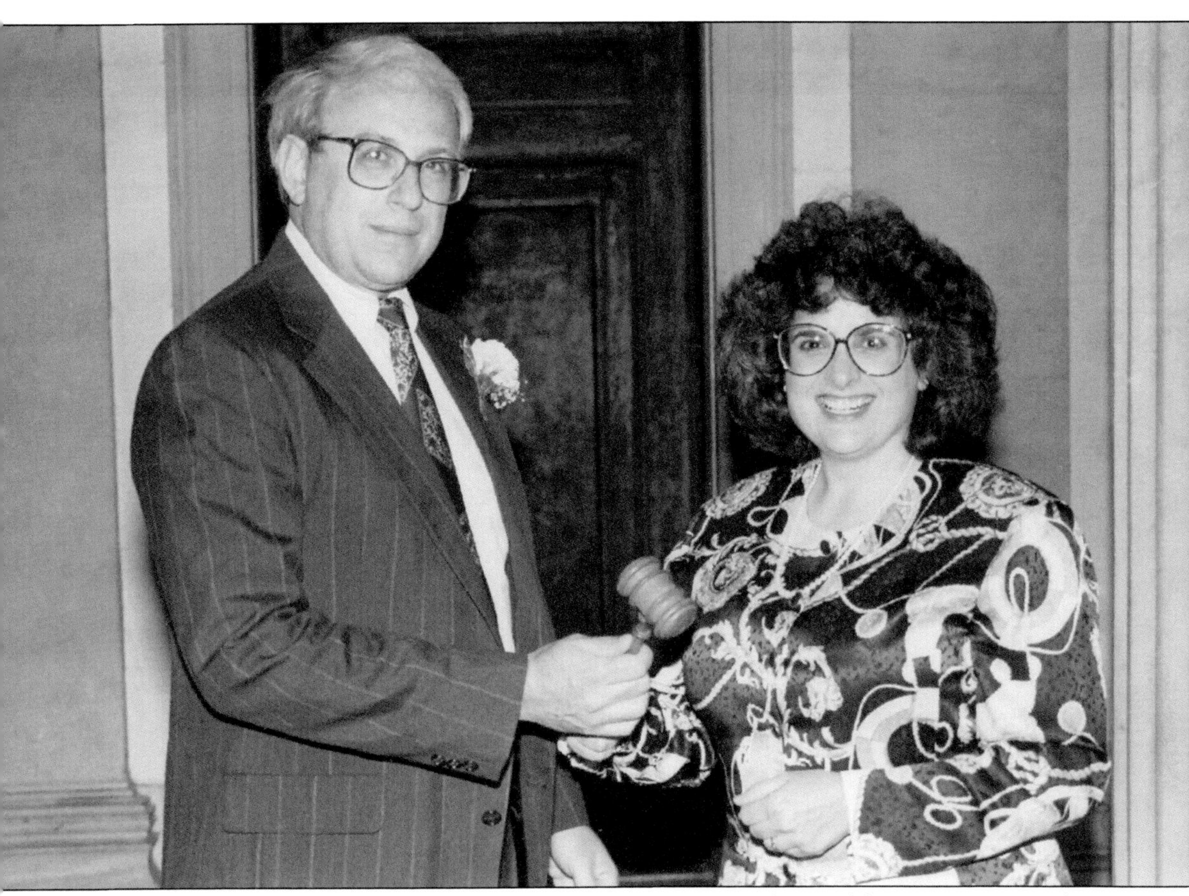

Dr. H. John Rubinstein, Medical Society president in 1992, accepts the gavel from outgoing president Dr. Amy Early. Each year, through the installation of officer process, the outgoing president of the Medical Society passes the gavel in a symbolic relay of leadership to the incoming president.

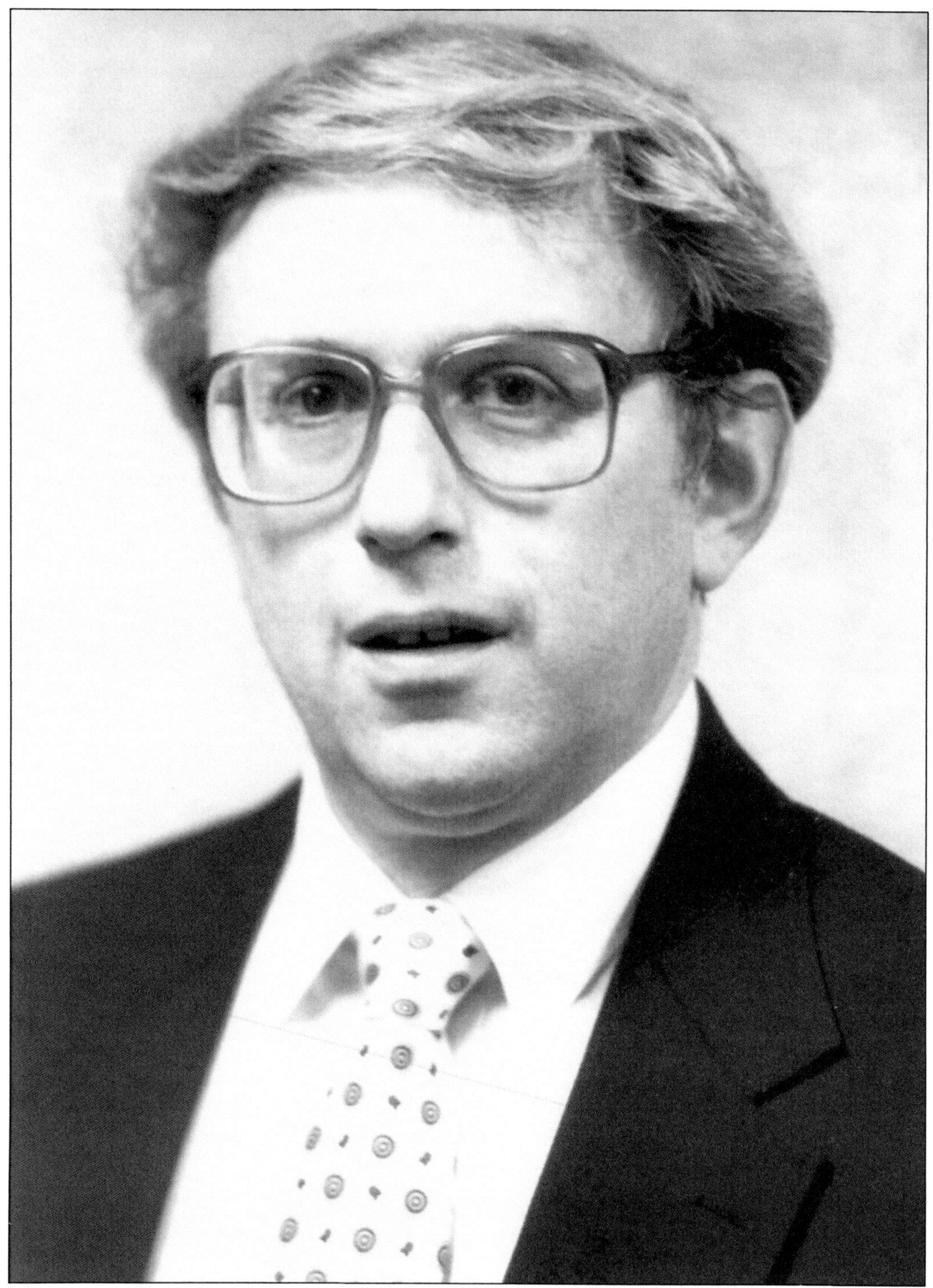

Dr. H. John Rubinstein, renowned Buffalo surgeon, was president of the Medical Society in 1992 and past president of the Western New York Chapter of the American College of Surgeons. During his tenure, Dr. Rubinstein posed questions about health care reform that are still significant today and asked poignant questions about the viability of a national health care system.

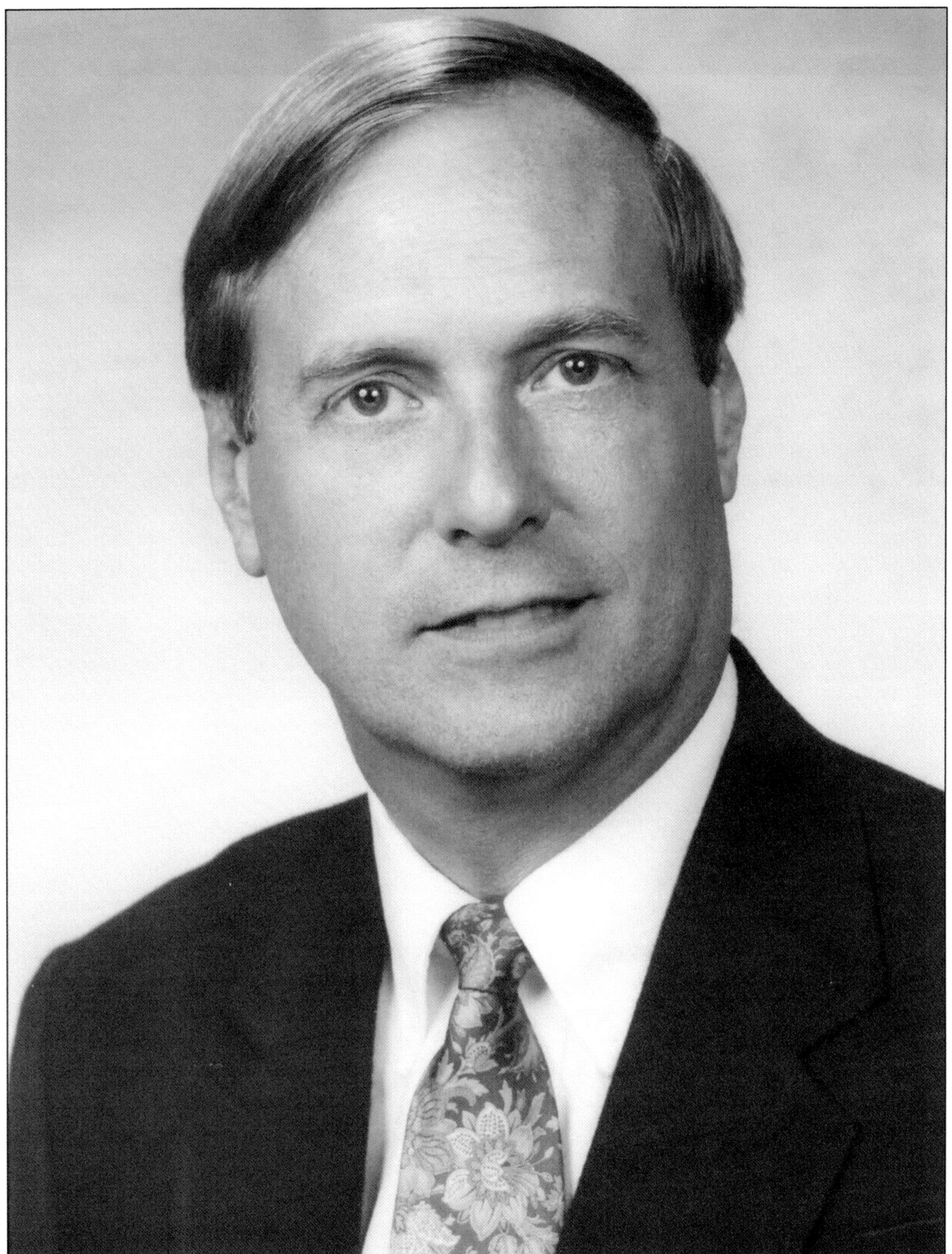

Dr. Richard Peer was founder and the first president of the Western New York Physicians Executive Group and president of the Buffalo Academy of Medicine, Buffalo Surgical Society, and Western New York Vascular Society. Dr. Peer has represented the state of New York as a delegate to the American Medical Association and was a founding member of the Kaleida Health Foundation Board. Dr. Peer was on the AMA Council on Long Range Planning and Development from 2005 to 2013 and served as vice chairman and then chairman from 2010 to 2012.

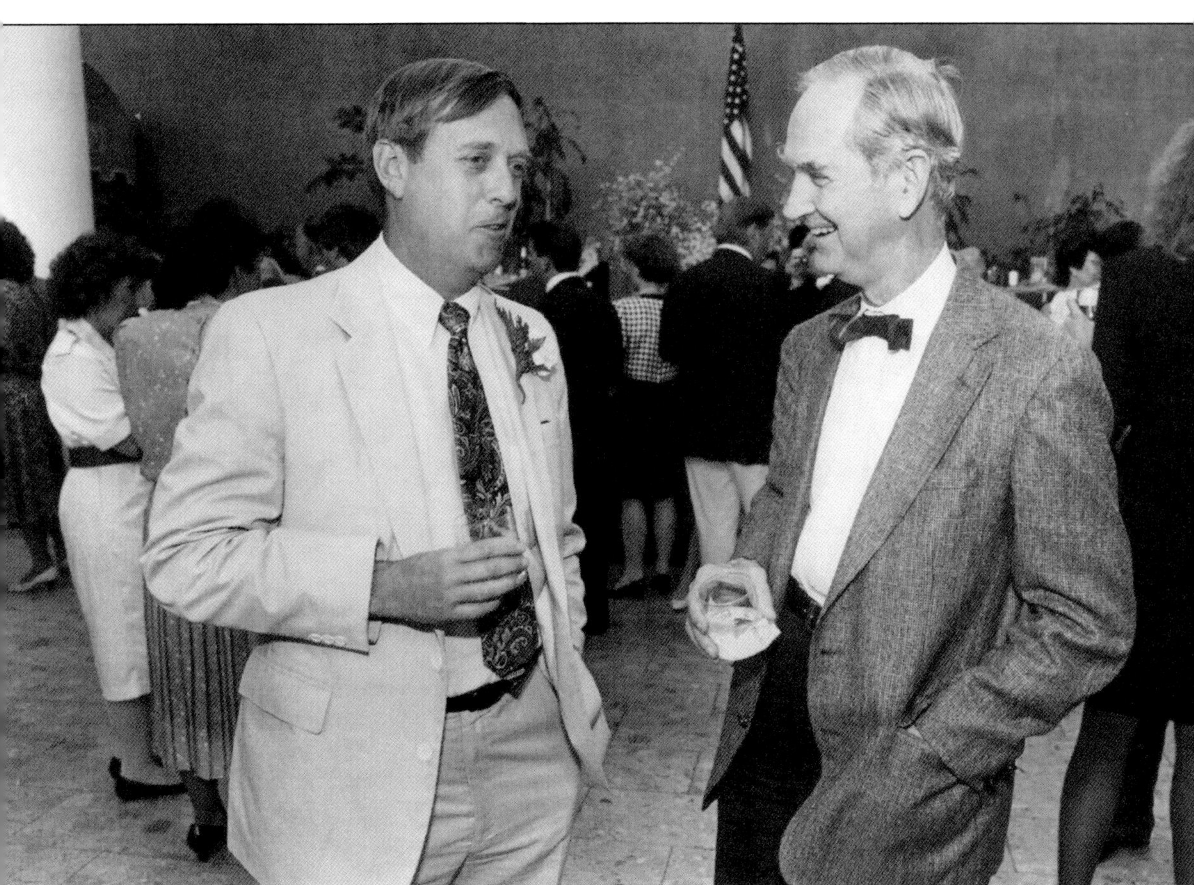

Dr. Richard Peer (left), Medical Society president in 1993, and Medical Society of the State of New York (MSSNY) president in 1996, is pictured with Dr. Charles Sherman, who served as president of the Monroe County Medical Society in 1965. Dr. Peer was MSSNY's 200th president and was a well-regarded surgeon in Buffalo. He received the Charles D. Sherman MD Student Award from MSSNY in 2013 for extraordinary assistance, availability, and support of the medical students' section of MSSNY throughout the state, and has served on the MLMIC Insurance Company board since 1998. From 2008 to 2018, he was vice president and corporate secretary of MLMIC and paved the way in liability reform at both the county and state level. Dr. Peer practices actively today, serving as the medical director of the Vascular Lab at Millard Fillmore Suburban Hospital and at Buffalo Medical Group.

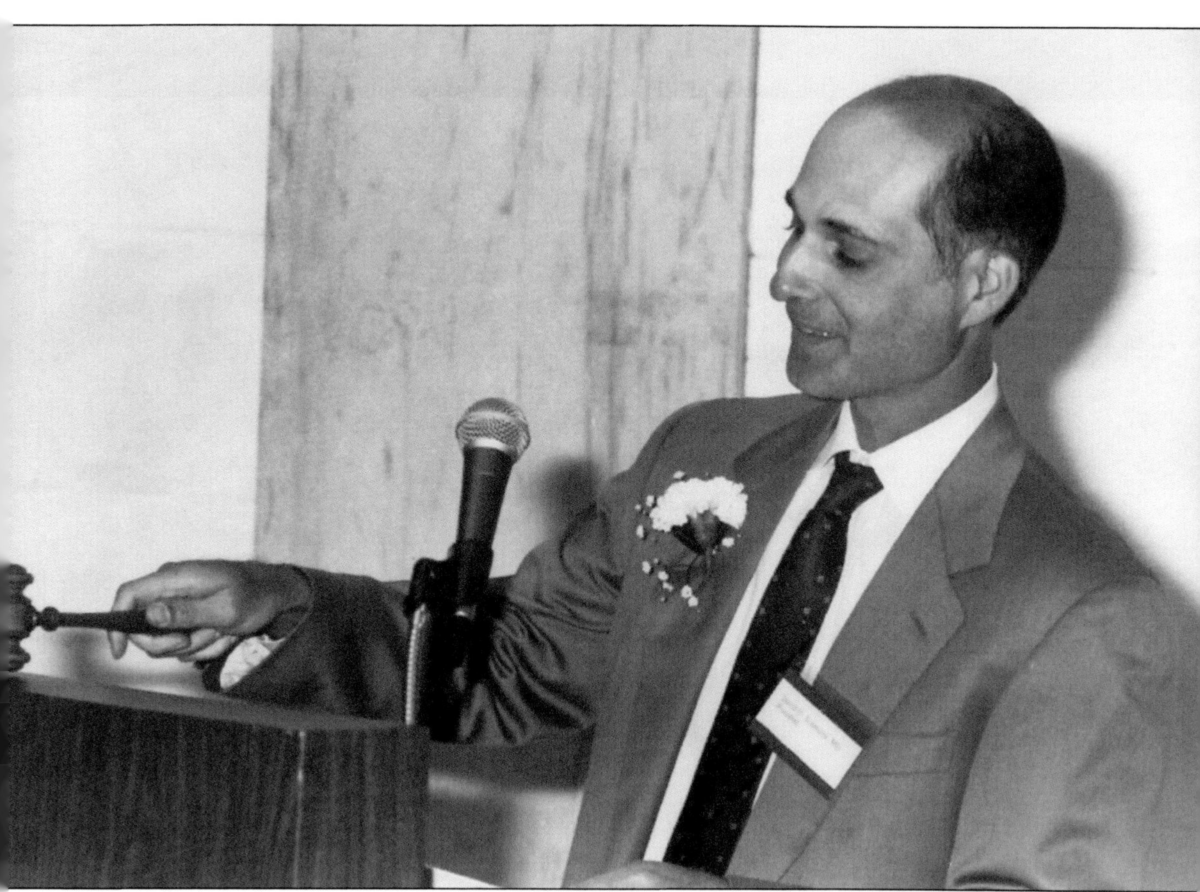

Dr. David Scamurra, Medical Society president in 1994, is seen here with gavel in hand calling to open the annual meeting at the Albright Knox Gallery on June 1, 1995. Dr. Scamurra is a board-certified pathologist and licensed to practice medicine in New York, Florida, and South Carolina.

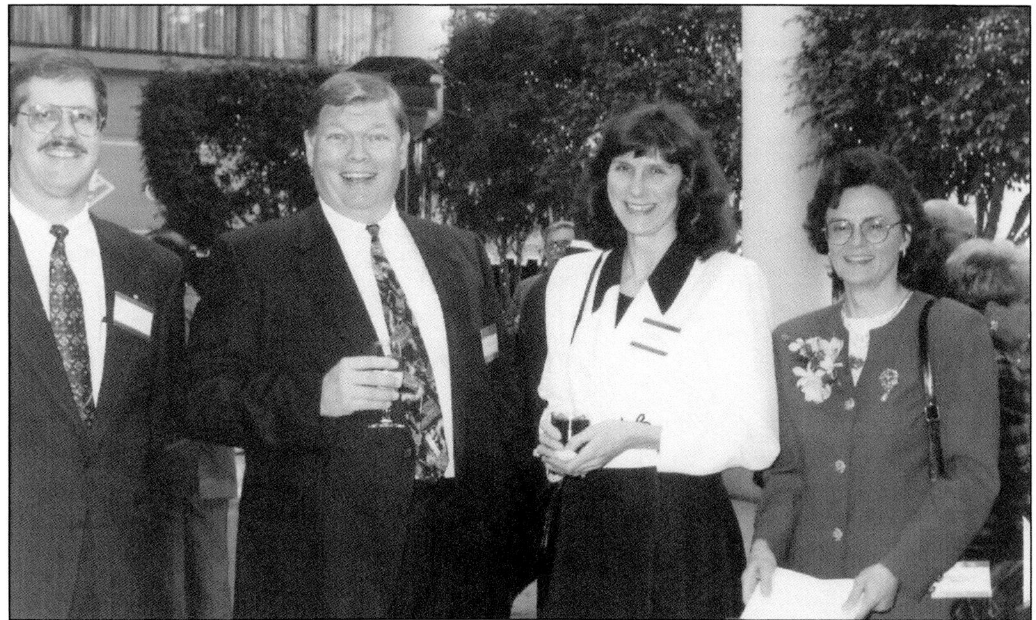

Dr. Evan Evans (second from left) is pictured here with Irene Snow, MD (far right), 1995 Medical Society president. Also pictured are Dr. Evans's wife, Sue Evans, and Dr. Snow's husband, John Herzig. A native of Binghamton, Dr. Snow came to Buffalo in 1977 for medical school, turning down an opportunity to interview at Johns Hopkins University.

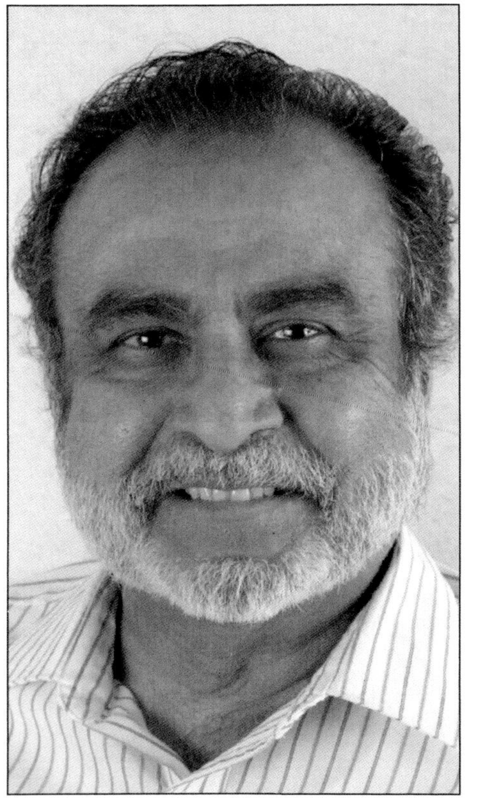

Dr. Sateesh K. Satchidanand is a longstanding member of the Medical Society. He was chairman of the Medical Services Committee (2009–2011) and teller of elections (1998–2018). He also served as. a delegate to the MSSNY for the past two years. Dr. Satchidanand graduated from Gandhi Medical College in Hyderabad, India, in 1967. He moved to the United Kingdom, where he trained for two years in pathology. He then completed the residency training program at SUNY at Buffalo Medical School in 1975. He joined the staff of Buffalo General Hospital and SUNYAB in 1976 and served as chief of anatomic pathology from 1985 to 1990. Dr. Satchidanand volunteered several years at the Buffalo Zoo helping the resident veterinarian in the diagnosis and treatment of diseases of animals. He also helped in conducting and supervising autopsies. Currently, he specializes in GI and liver pathology and teaches at SUNYAB and is on the staff at Sisters of Charity Hospital and Kenmore Mercy Hospital. Dr. Satchidanand is a fellow of the College of American Pathologists and has been a member of the House of Delegates representing New York since 2004. He resides in Tonawanda with his wife, Yashodhara Satchidanand, a retired palliative physician.

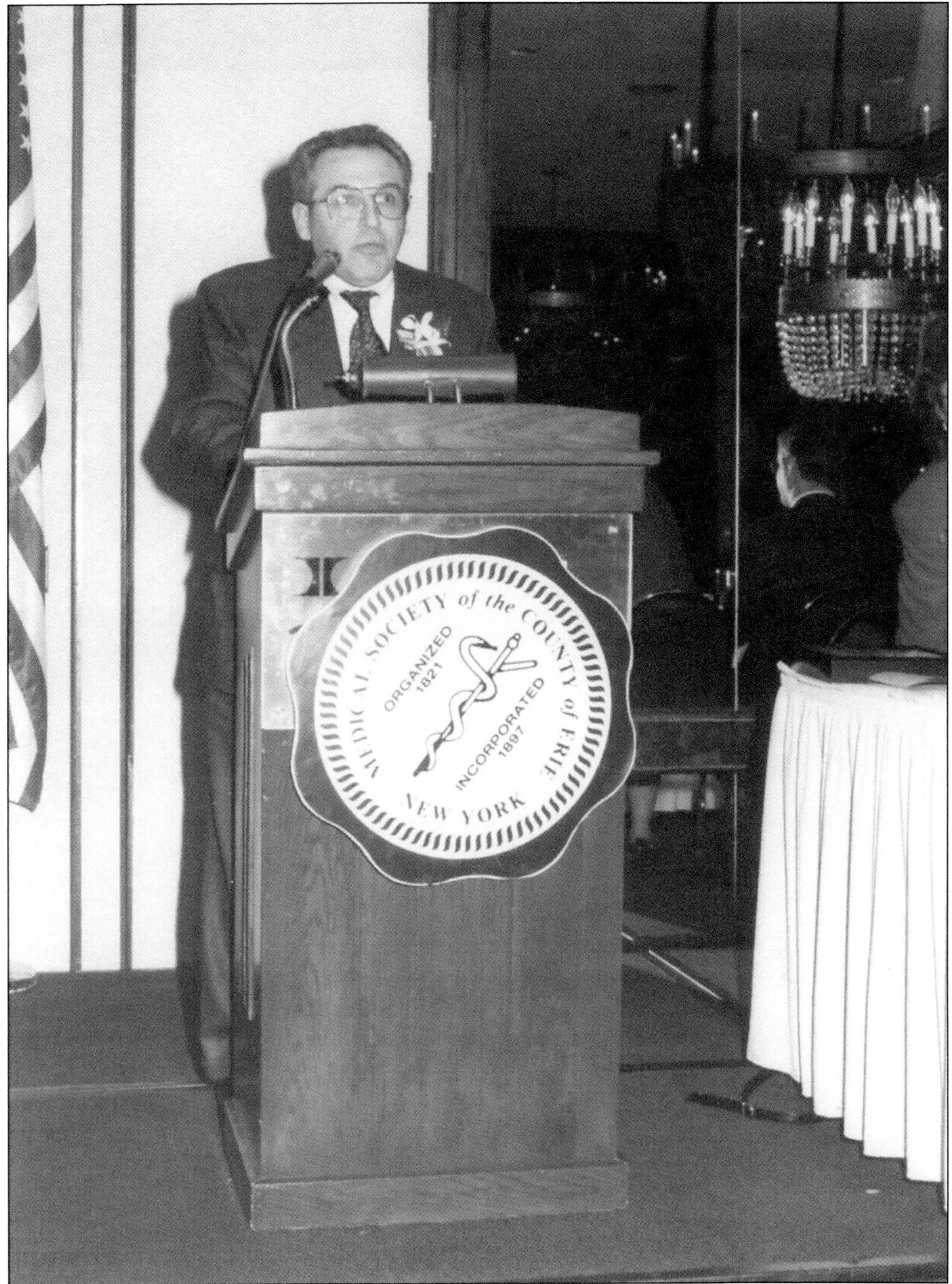

Russell Bessette, MD, DDS, was president of the Medical Society in 1996–1997. He served as clinical professor of surgery at the University at Buffalo School of Medicine and established a new state agency—the New York State Office of Science, Technology, and Academic Research—that supported over $1.3 billion in peer-reviewed research grants and stimulated $12.8 billion in university research and development.

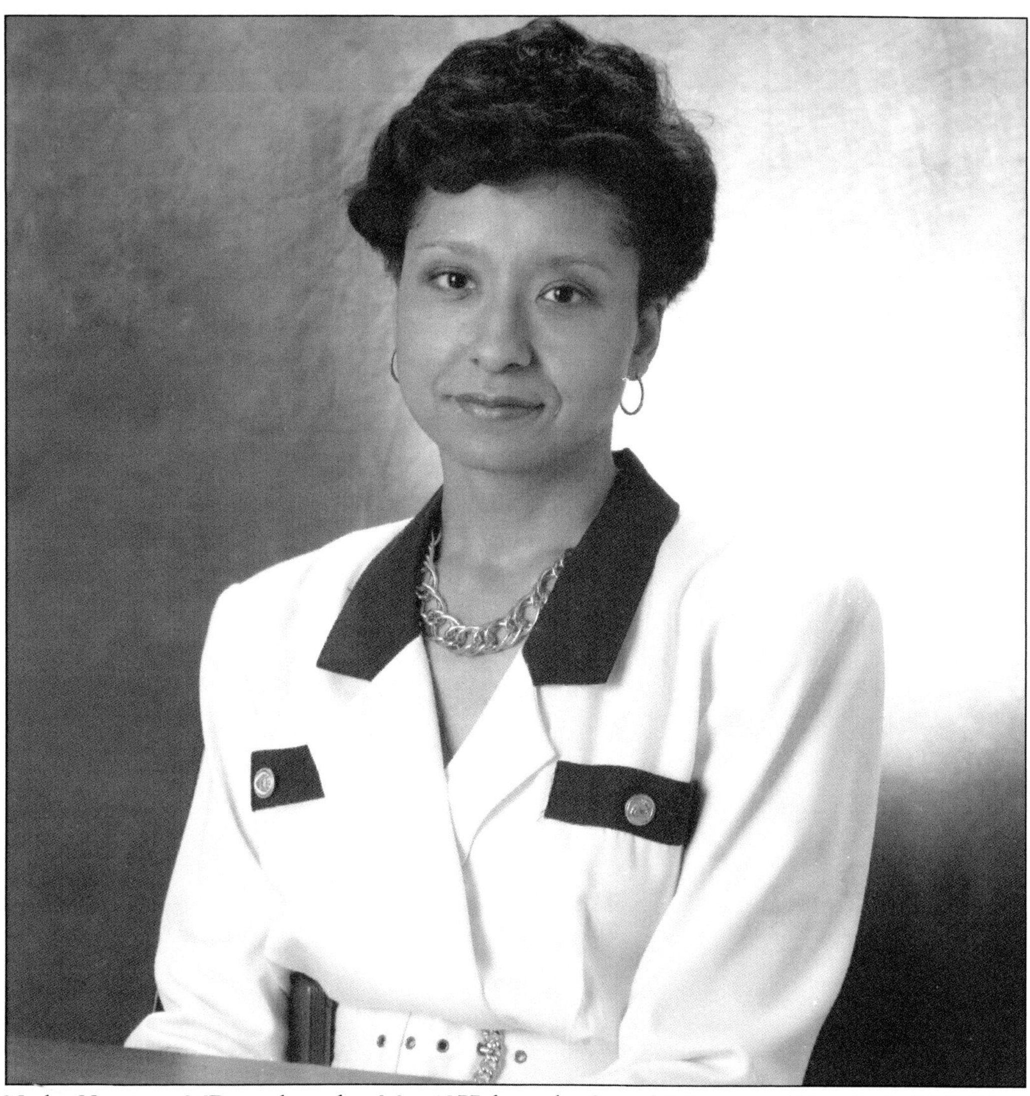

Nedra Harrison, MD, graduated in May 1977 from the State University of New York (SUNY) at Buffalo and completed her general surgery internship and residency training at Millard Fillmore Hospital in Buffalo from 1977 to 1982. Dr. Harrison was licensed in New York state in 1979 and joined the Medical Society of Erie County in 1980. She was the first woman to be elected president of the University at Buffalo Medical Alumni Association. Dr. Harrison became the first and only African American female to serve as president of the Medical Society of Erie County (1998). Among her many awards, she has received the American Medical Association's Physicians Recognition Award and the Daemen College Distinguished Alumni Award. She now practices in Scottsdale, Arizona, and was named to *Phoenix* magazine's Top Doctors list in 2011.

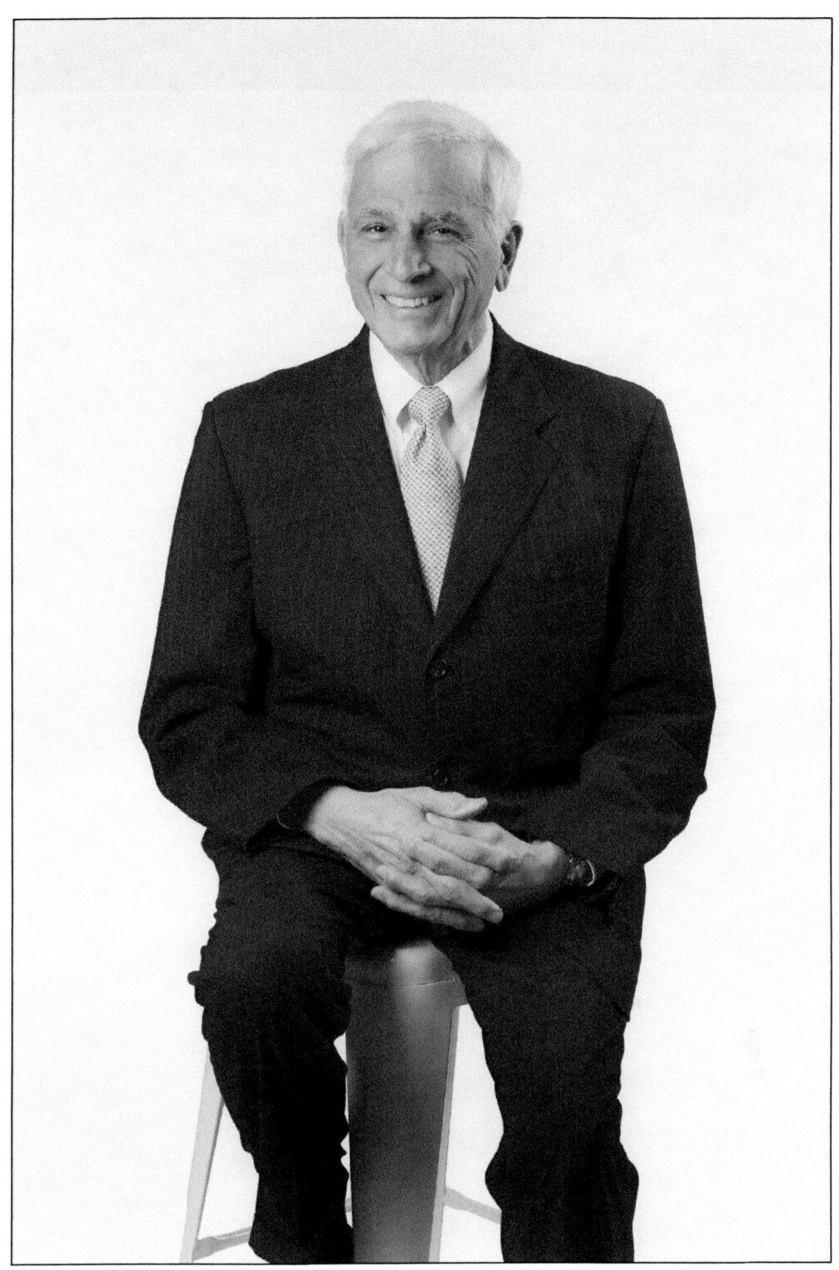

Dr. Thomas Lombardo is a board-certified orthopedic surgeon with over 40 years of experience. His practice these days is non-surgical, but he acts as a consultant to Excelsior Orthopaedics. His passions for eliminating pain and helping people have led him to a long, rewarding career of making sure thousands of patients return to normalcy. Dr. Lombardo and his wife, Donna, have been married for over 50 years and raised four daughters. His life today centers around his family. After decades in the operating room, he now tries to spend as much time outside as possible. Dr. Lombardo served as president of the Western New York Orthopaedic Society in 1985, president of the New York State Society of Orthopaedic Surgeons in 2000–2001, and sat on the New York State Society of Orthopaedic Surgeons Board of Directors from 1985 to 2017. Dr. Lombardo served as president of the Medical Society of Erie County in 2013 and has been a member for 41 years.

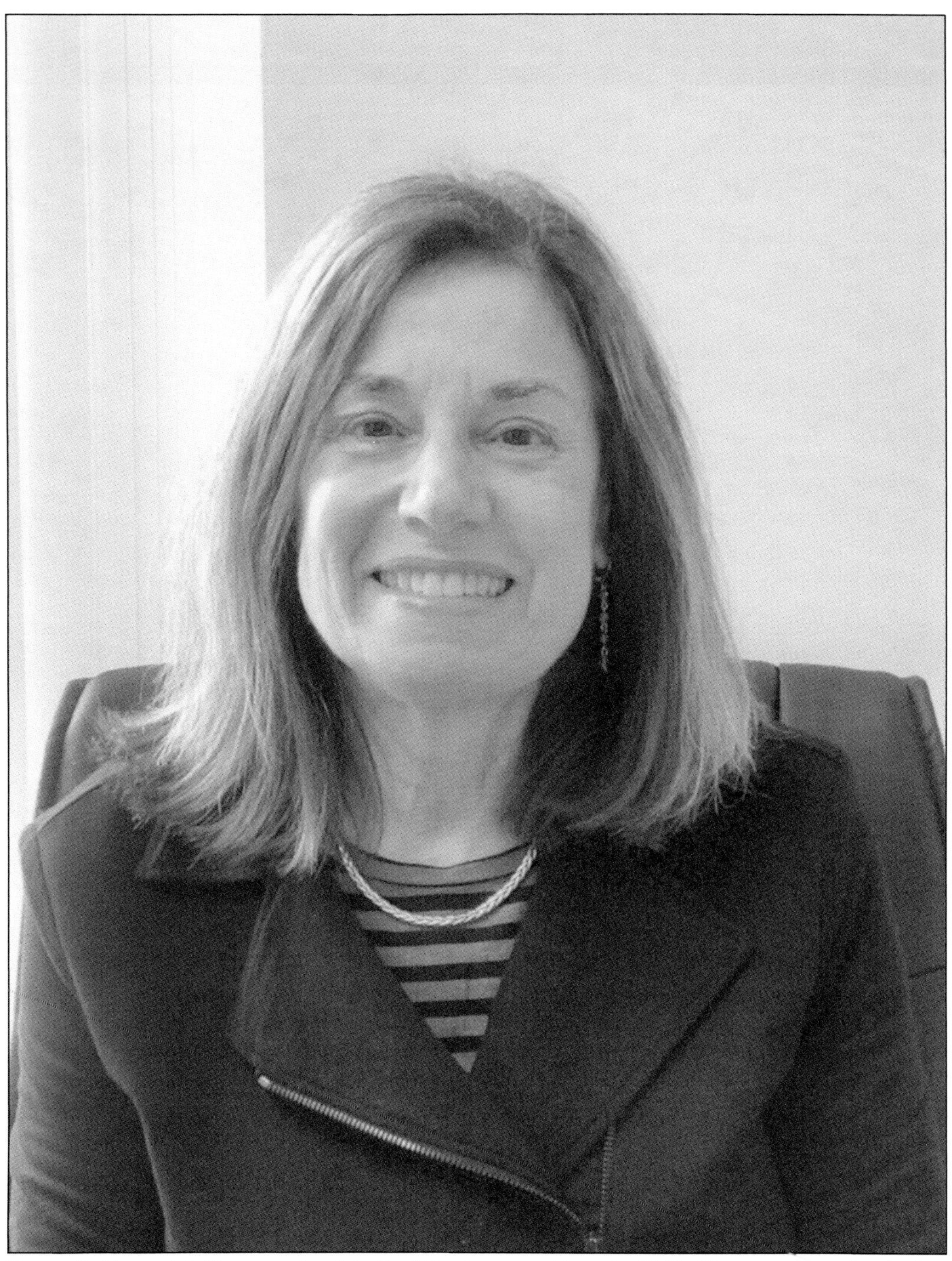

Susan Baldassari, MD, served as Medical Society president in 2001. She was one of only five female presidents at the Medical Society when she held that seat in 2001. Dr. Baldassari is an internal medicine physician and practices today in Amherst, New York.

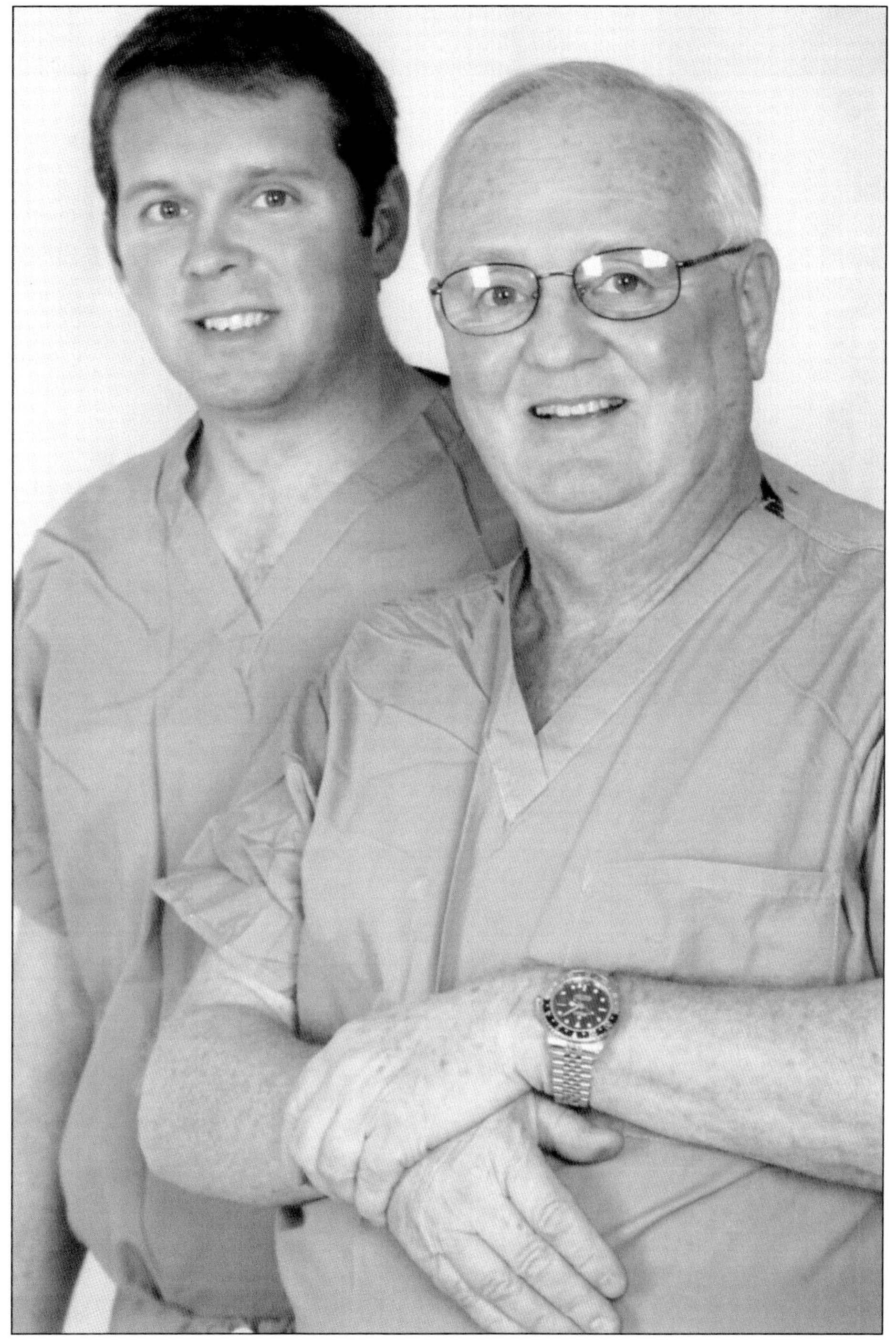

Pictured here in 2007 are Dr. Kenneth Eckhert III (left), Medical Society president in 2019–2020, and his father, Dr. Kenneth Eckhert Jr., president in 2004–2005.

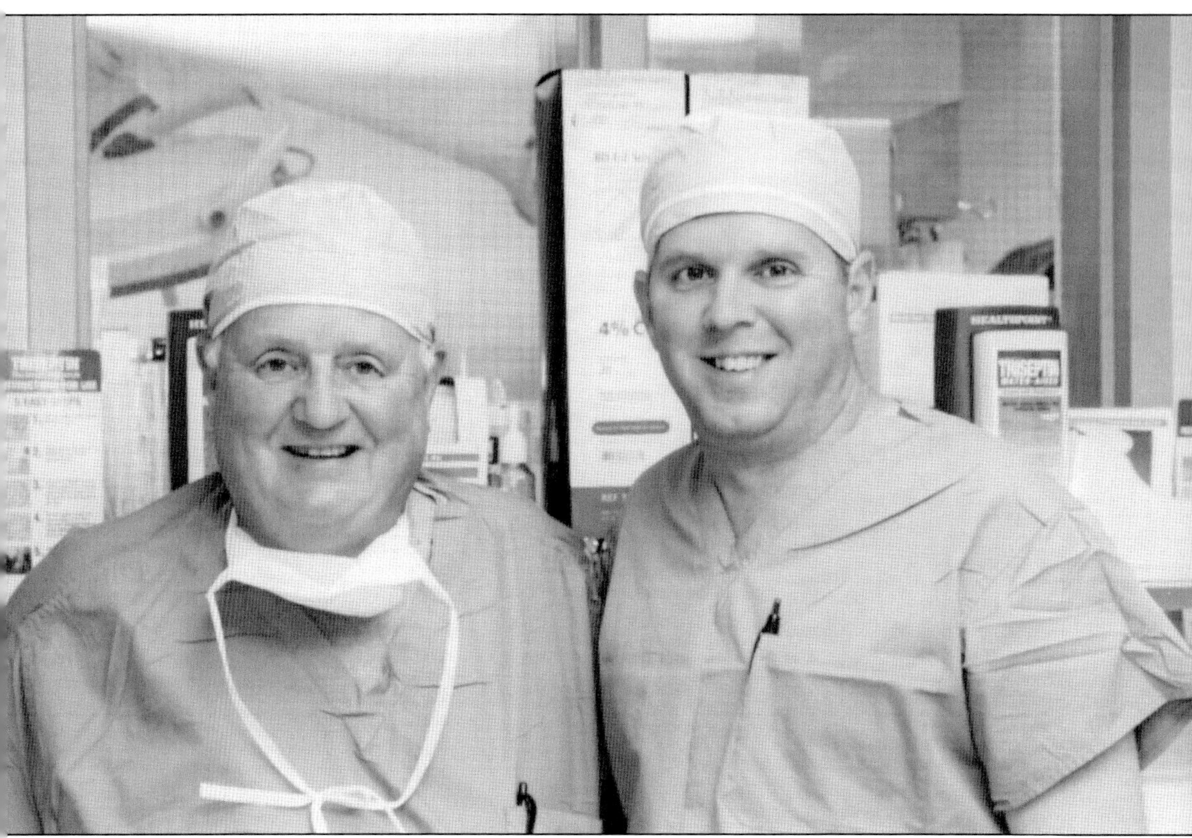

Pictured here are Dr. Kenneth Eckhert Jr. (left) and Dr. Kenneth Eckhert III at Buffalo Children's Hospital in 2010 when they worked together as attendings. Like his father and grandfather, Dr. Eckhert III serves as a board-certified general surgeon, specializing in general laparoscopic and robotic surgery.

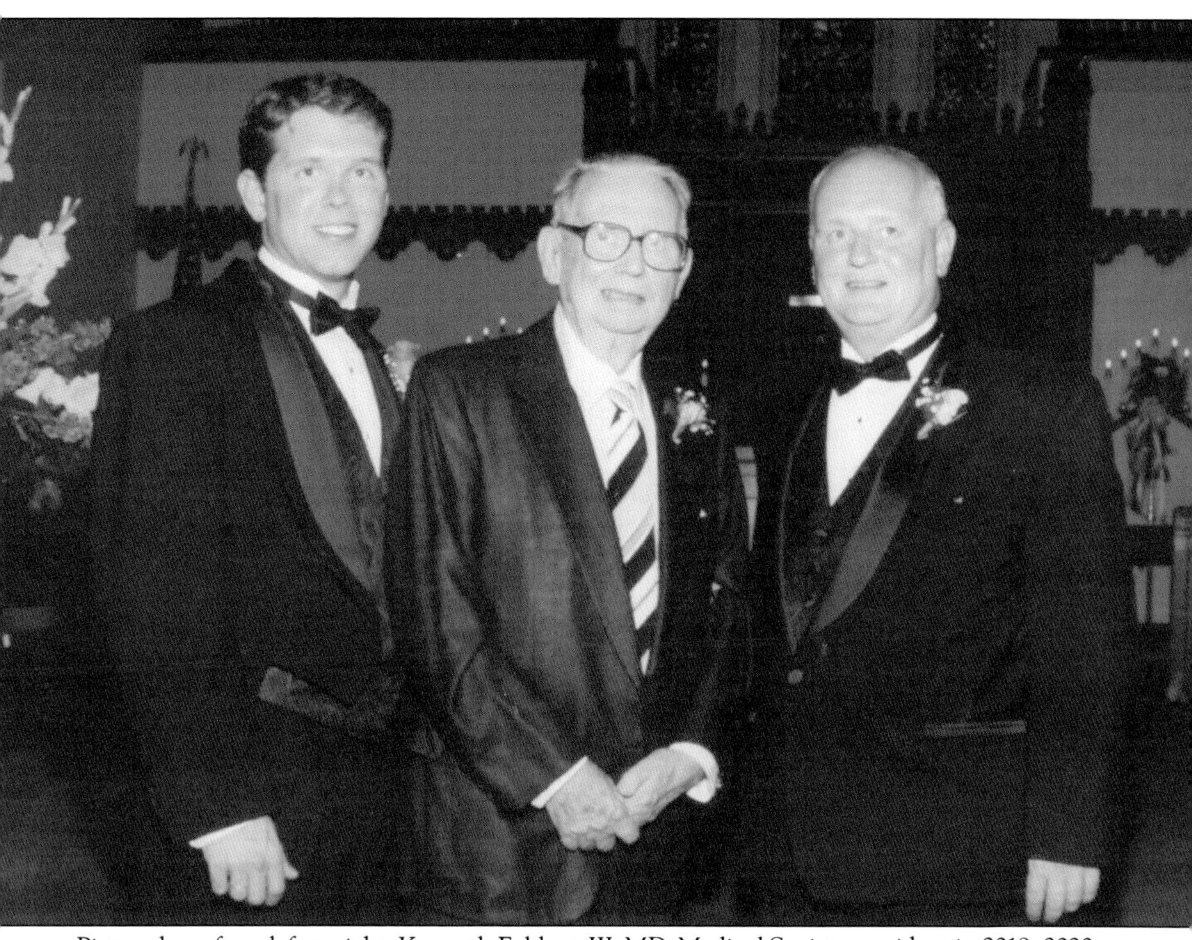

Pictured are, from left to right, Kenneth Eckhert III, MD, Medical Society president in 2019–2020; his grandfather Kenneth Eckhert, MD, president in 1960–1961; and Dr. Kenneth Eckhert Jr., president in 2004–2005. The Eckhert family is the only family to have spanned three generations as presidents in the 200-year history of the Medical Society of Erie County.

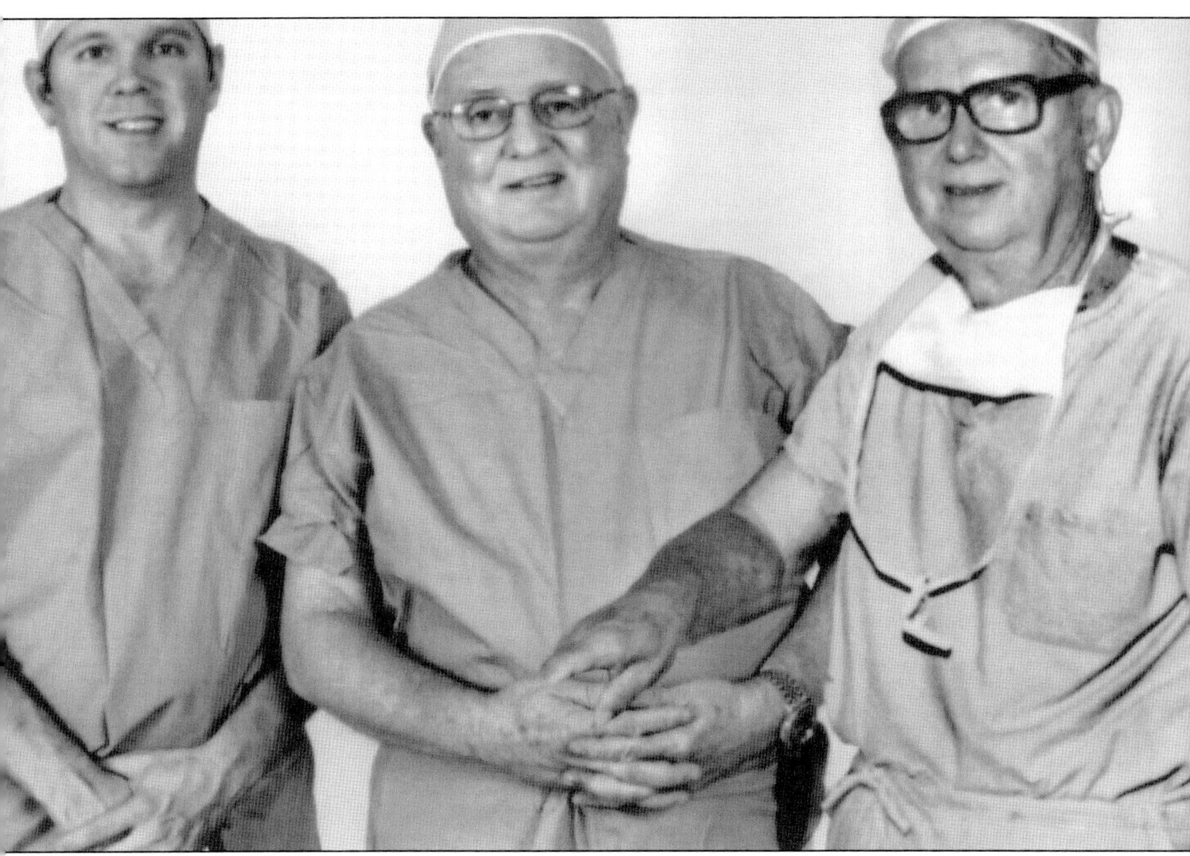

Pictured are, from left to right, Dr. Kenneth Eckhert III, Dr. Kenneth Eckhert Jr., and Dr. Kenneth Eckhert. Dr. Kenneth Eckhert set into motion a longstanding leadership tradition in his family. He was appointed as only the 13th cochairman by Gov. Nelson Rockefeller for the regional planning committee created in preparation for the 1971 White House Conference on Aging. Dr. Eckhert received the prestigious 1997 Clara Barton Volunteer of the Year Award for his service at the Red Cross.

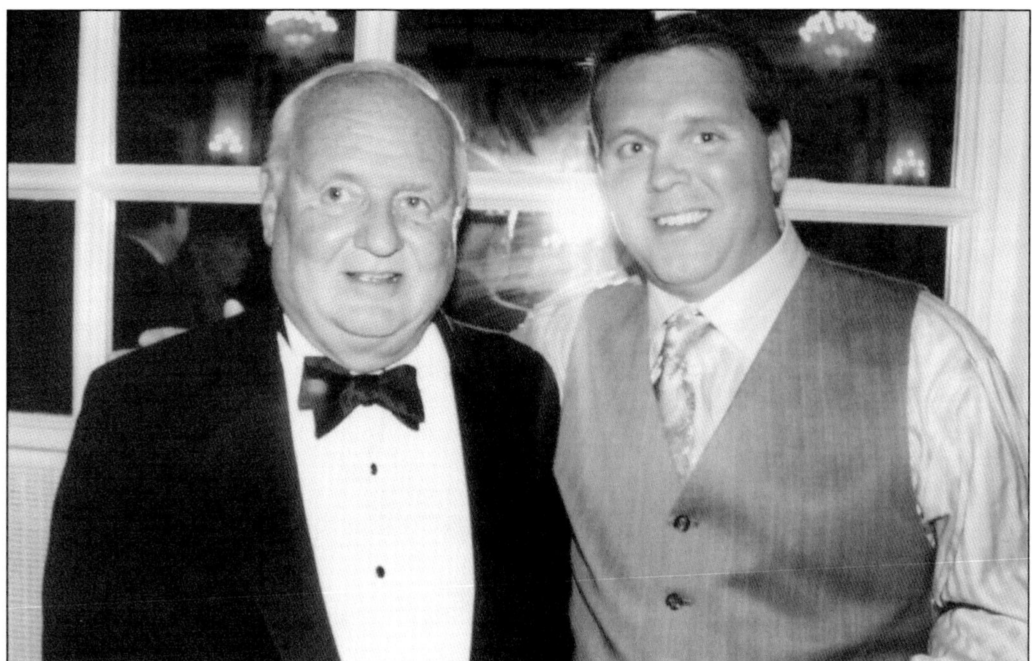

Seen here in 2009 are Dr. Kenneth Eckhert Jr. (left) and his son Kenneth Eckhert III, MD. Dr. Eckhert Jr. earned his master's degree from the University of West Virginia in 1964 and his medical degree from the University at Buffalo in 1968. Dr. Eckhert Jr. served as commanding officer for the New York State Air National Guard from 1973 to 1977, director of the Children's Hospital/Kaleida Breast Cancer Center in 2002, and taught as adjunct clinical professor of surgery at the University at Buffalo School of Medicine.

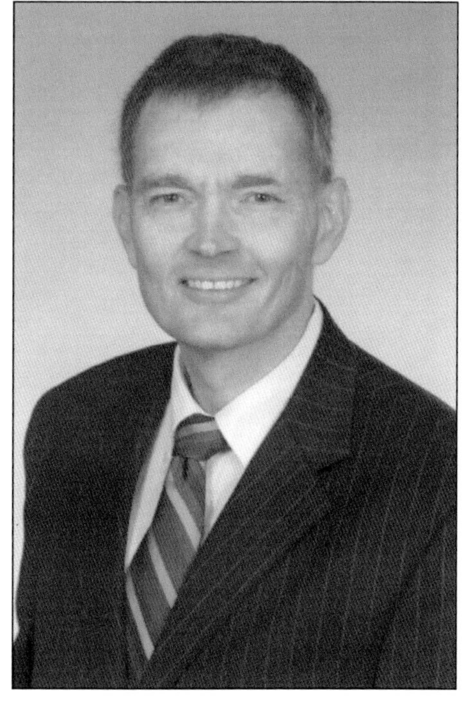

Thomas J. Madejski, MD, was president of the Orleans County Medical Society and the Medical Society of the State of New York (2018), where he served as president, vice president, and treasurer, and as commissioner of socio-medical economics and vice-chair of the Legislative and Physician Advocacy committee. He has represented New York in the American Medical Association House of Delegates for the past 15 years and was elected to the Council of Medical Service in 2015 and the board of trustees in 2020. In 2019, he was named to the Health Care Power 50 list by City & State magazine. Dr. Madejski graduated from the School of Pharmacy, SUNY at Buffalo, and the School of Medicine, SUNY Health Science Center in Syracuse. Dr. Madejski currently serves as chief of medicine at Medina Memorial Hospital and as medical director at The Villages of Orleans Health and Rehabilitation Center in Albion, New York, and is a clinical instructor in medicine at the University of Rochester and a clinical instructor in pharmacy at the University of Buffalo. Dr. Madejski resides in Albion with his wife, Sandra.

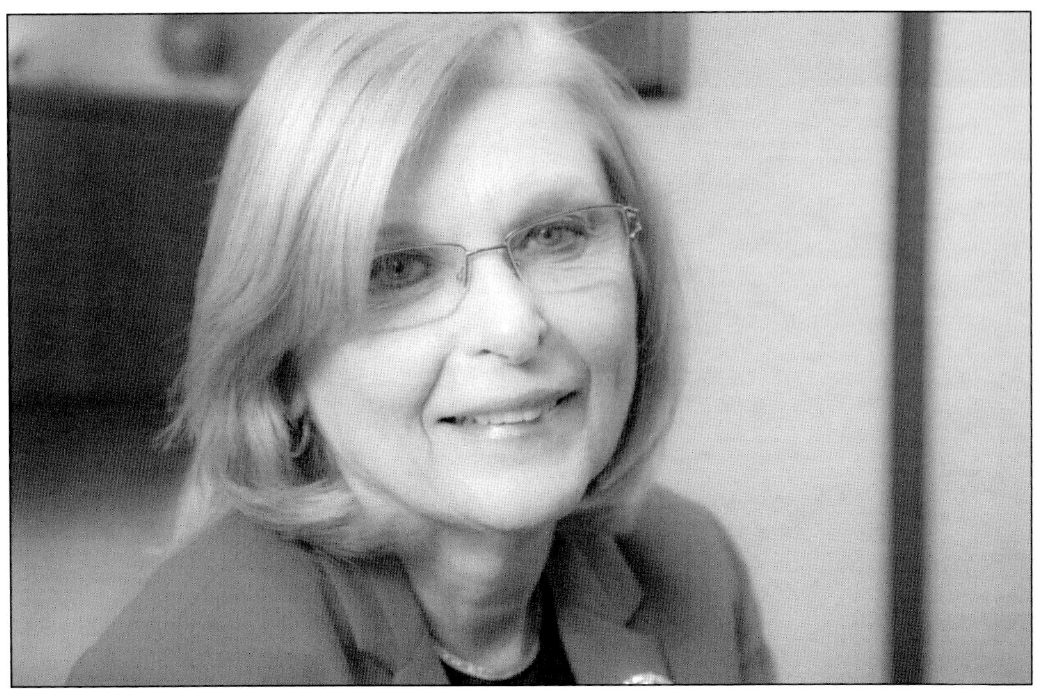

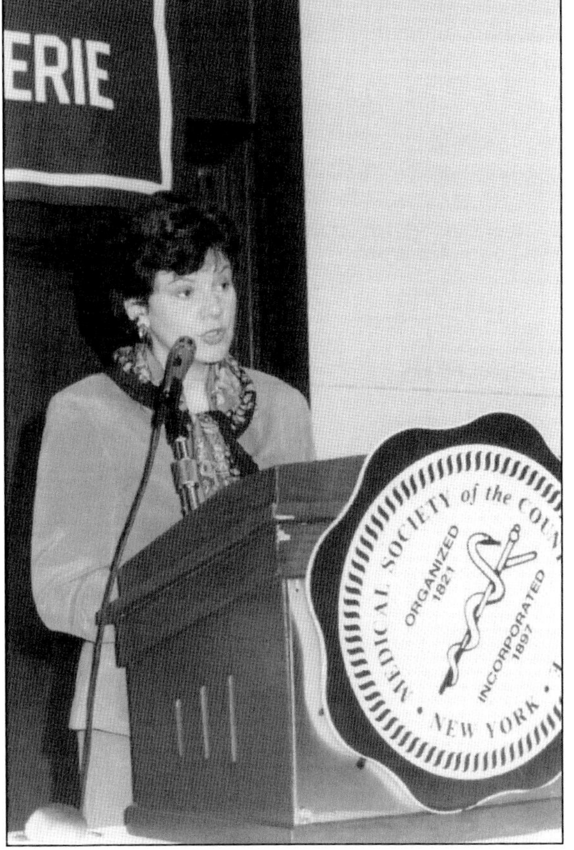

Christine Nadolny, successor to Richard Trecasse and predecessor to Aimana ElBahtity, served as executive director of the Medical Society of Erie County. Nadolny spent 24 years at the Medical Society, 20 of which were in the role of executive director. She was awarded the Medical Executive Lifetime Achievement Award by the American Medical Association in 2017. Nadolny retired on July 1, 2020, and lives in Orchard Park, New York, with her husband, Ronald.

In May 2005, the Centers for Disease Control and Prevention honored Medical Society keynote speaker Dr. Barbara DeBuono as one of five public health heroes nationwide. In 2011, she was named president and CEO of Orbis International, a global health organization that prevents and treats blindness with transforming care to millions of families throughout the developing world.

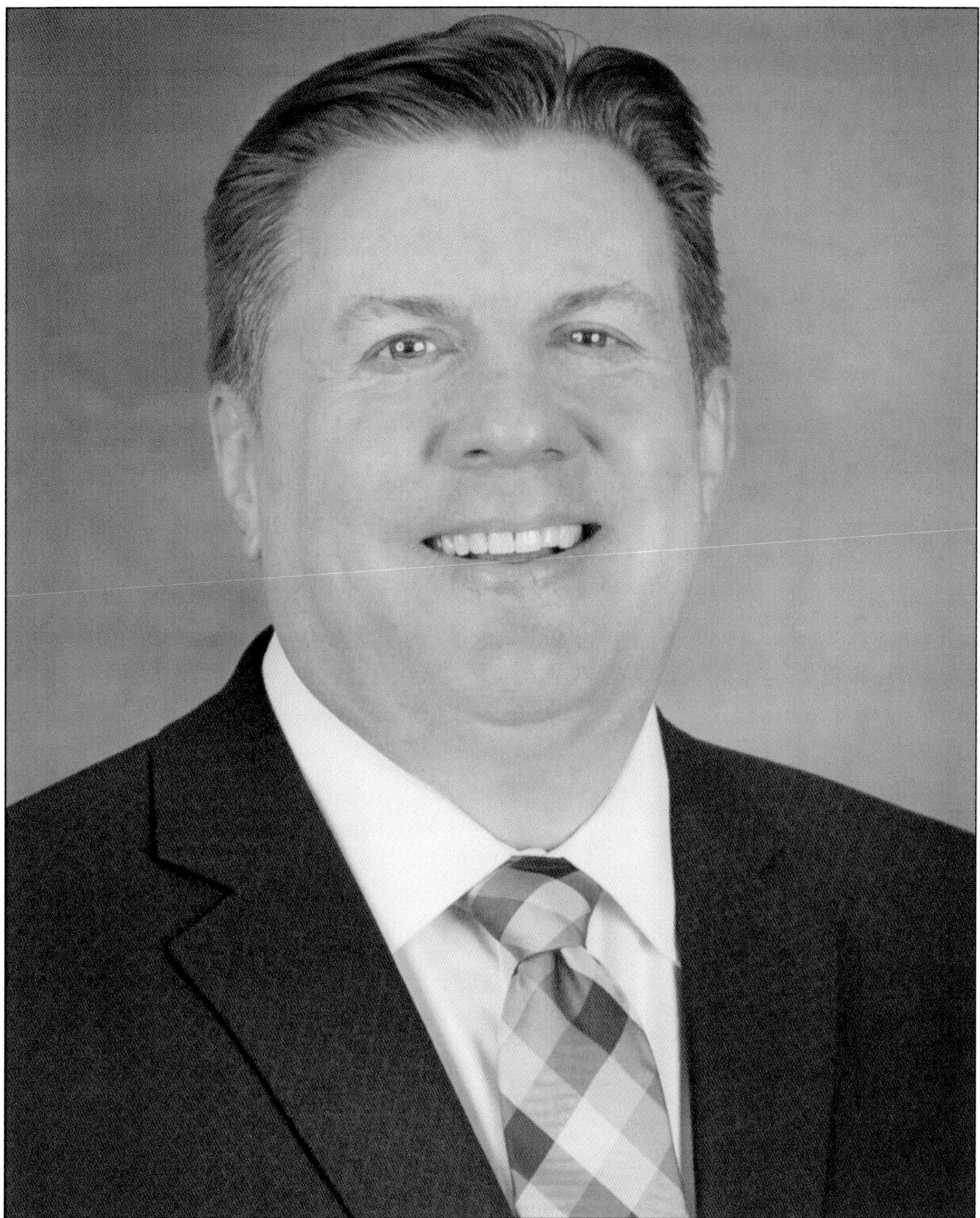

Richard Paul Vienne Jr., DO, served as president of the Medical Society of Erie County in 2005–2006 and was associate clinical professor of medicine at SUNY Buffalo School of Medicine. Dr. Vienne's countless professional and community achievements include his rising in the ranks in the Medical Society and his leadership at Boy Scout Troop No. 457. Dr. Vienne served on multiple committees, including Excellus/Univera's Drug Utilization Review, Healthcare Quality and Benefits Management, Adult QA, Obesity Initiative, and Medical Policy Committee. He also served as the Medical Society liaison to the Erie County Bar Association. Notably, Dr. Vienne also served as president of the advisory board for Houghton College and past president of the Greater Niagara Frontier Council of the Boys Scouts of America.

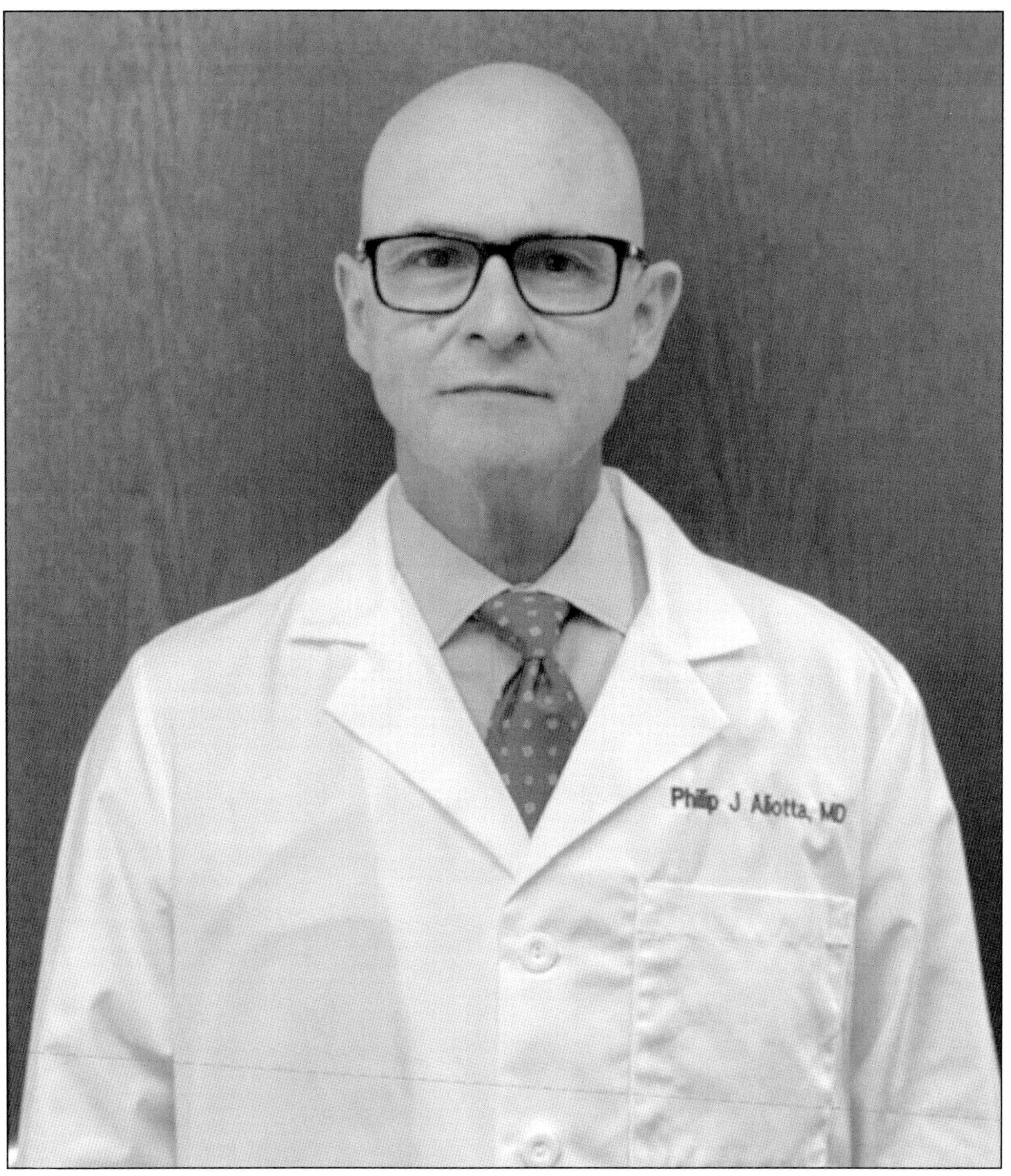

Dr. Philip Aliotta served as Medical Society president in 2006–2007. Dr. Aliotta, MD, MSHA, FASC, is a board-certified urologist. He graduated from the University at Buffalo School of Medicine in 1982 and earned his master's degree from the University of Colorado at Denver in 1994. He served as president of the Western New York Chapter of the American College of Surgeons from 1993 to 1995. Among his countless accomplishments, Dr. Aliotta served as instructor of urology at SUNY Buffalo. He was the medical director and founder of the Center for Urologic Research of Western New York, LLC.

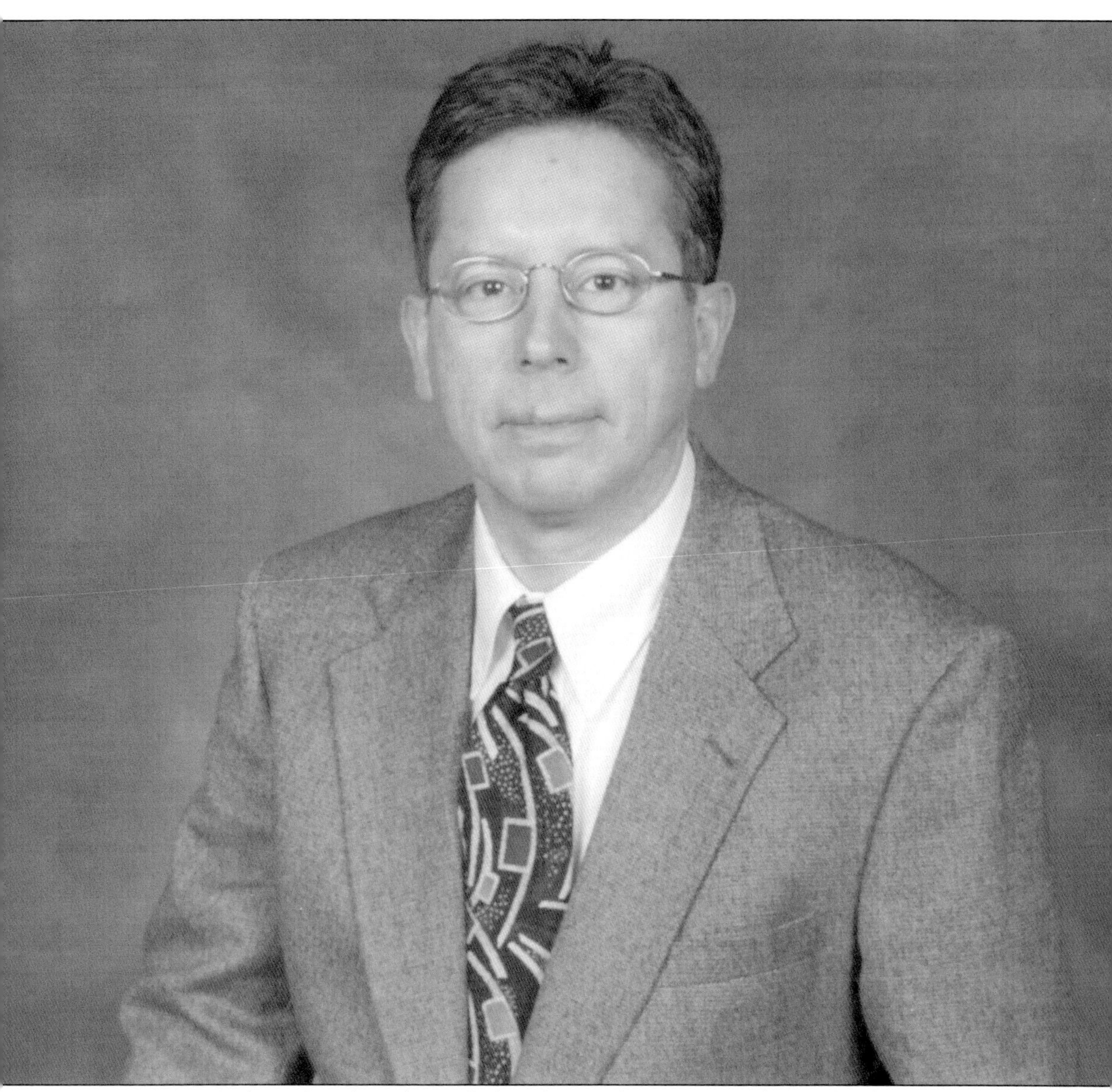

Ernesto Diaz-Ordaz, MD, a board-certified otolaryngologist, sits on the Medical Society of Erie County's board as a past president (2007). He served as president of the Buffalo Otolaryngological Society from 2002 to 2004. Dr. Diaz-Ordaz is a veteran of the US Navy, serving as commander in 1992. He has dedicated much time over the years as a society member, serving on multiple county Medical Society committees, several of MSSNY's committees, and as a member of MSSNY's House of Delegates.

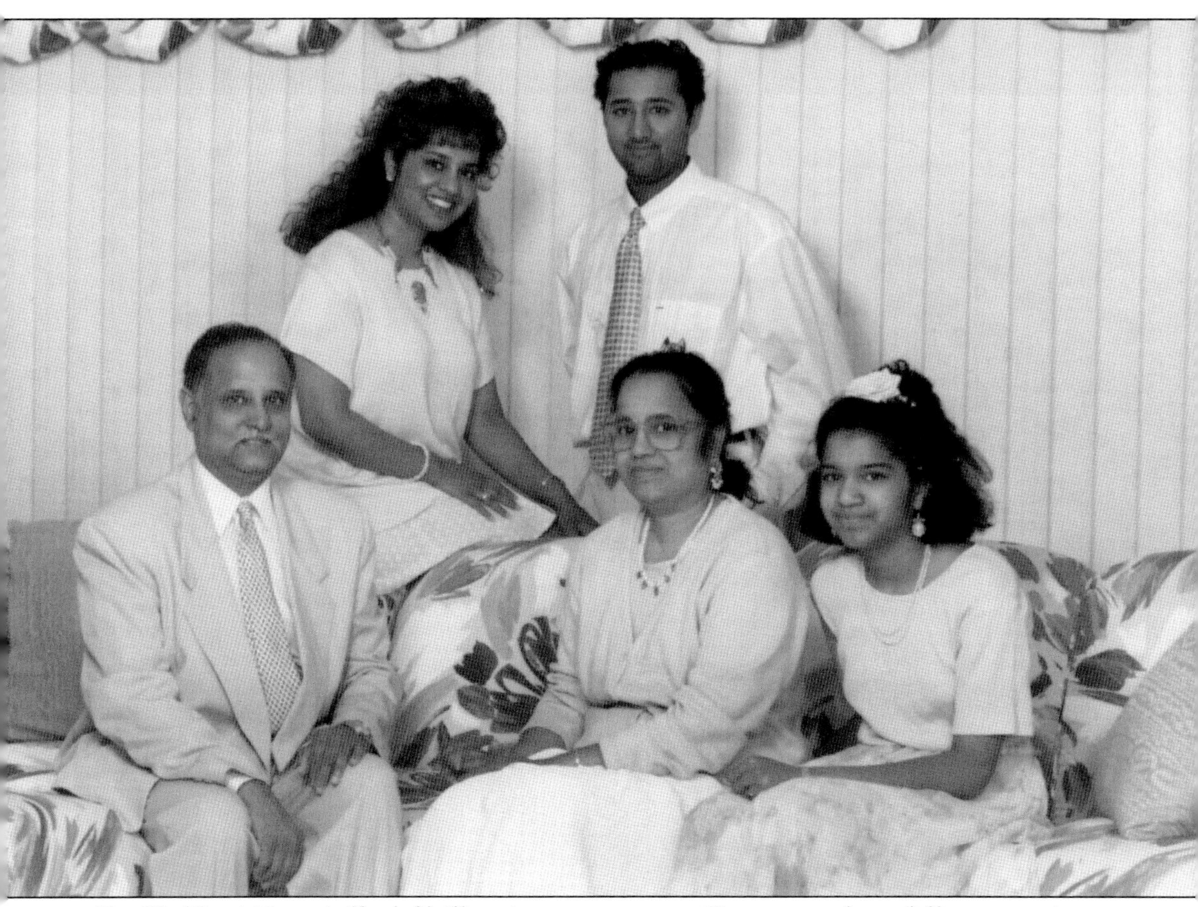

Dr. Chelikani Varma's (far left) illustrious career spans 57 years on three different continents (North America, Europe, and Asia). His medical specialty is pediatrics. He served as a clinical associate professor of pediatrics and on the board of admissions at the University at Buffalo School of Medicine. He was a director at St Joseph's Hospital and was employed at Millard Fillmore Suburban, Sisters of Charity Hospital, BryLin Hospital, St. Mary's Hospital, Erie County Medical Center, and Children's Hospital of Buffalo. Dr. Varma received numerous distinctions, including Women & Children's Hospital of Buffalo class of 2017 honoree, American Medical Association Physician's Recognition Award, Buffalo Pediatric Society's Distinguished Alumni Award, Children's Hospital of Buffalo Pediatric Residents' Association's Excellence in Teaching, Children's Hospital of Buffalo Pediatric Residents' Association's Frederick B. Wilkes Memorial Teaching Award, Outstanding Teacher Award by SUNY Buffalo (Department of Pediatrics), Medical Society of State of New York Service Award, and DLC Pediatrics as a Teaching Site for the medical students of the SUNY Buffalo School of Medicine. He also contributed to the Legal Guidelines for Medical Offices on behalf of the Liaison Committee of the Medical Society. Dr. Varma earned his medical degree from Kasturba Medical College Manipal in Mangalore, India, and his postgraduate degree in adolescent medicine in Lucknow, India. He completed his medical residencies at National Health Service in England and National Health Service in Wales, Mercy Hospital, and Children's Hospital of Buffalo. He also earned his private pilot's license at the age of 15.

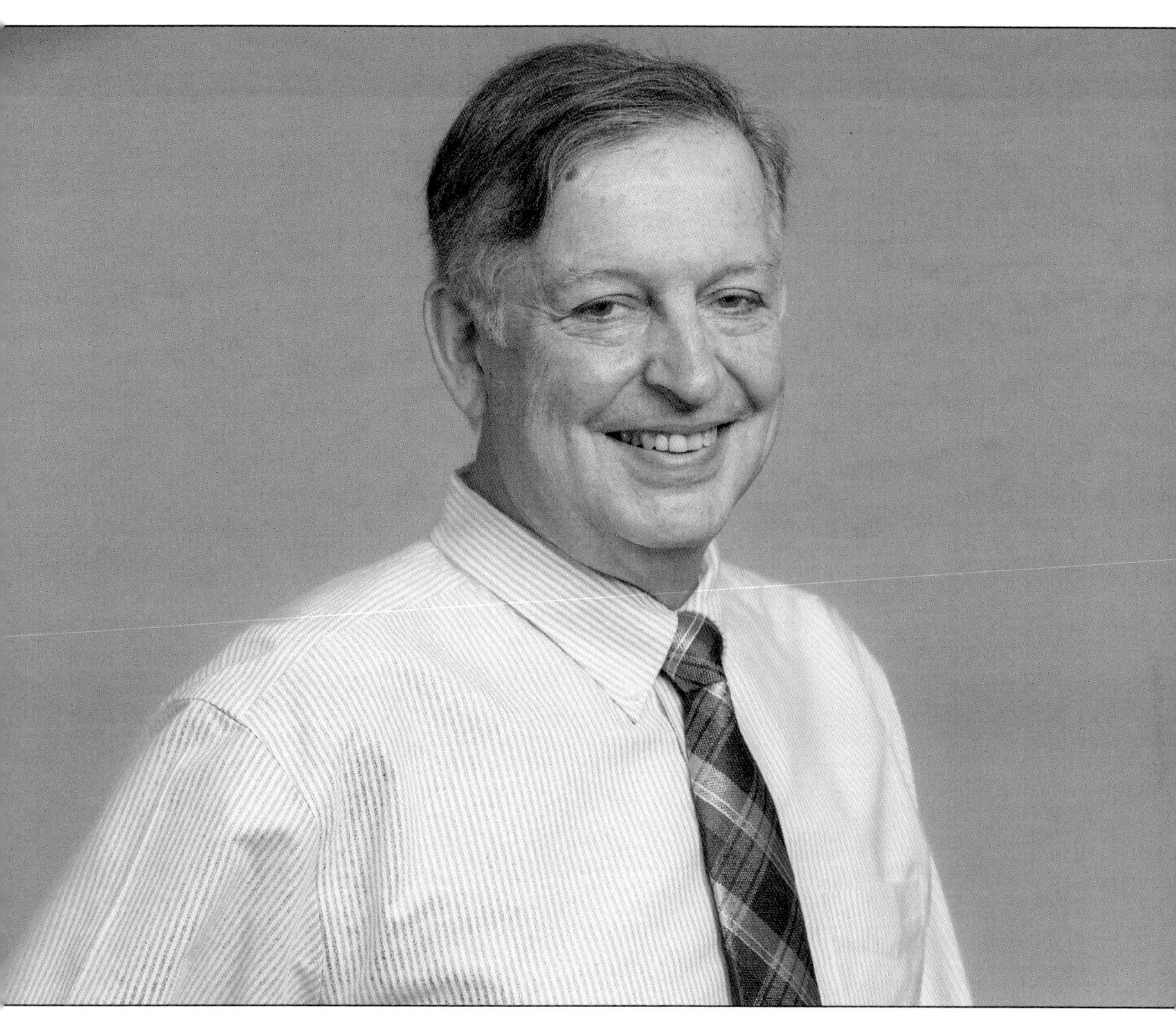

Dr. Edward Kelly Bartels served as president of the Medical Society in 2008–2009. He attended the University at Buffalo School of Medicine from 1976 to 1980 and completed his residency at the University of Rochester in 1984. Dr. Bartels served as the president of the medical staff at Sisters of Charity Hospital in 1995 and sat on Catholic Health System's OB/GYN Quality Improvement Committee. Dr. Bartels joined his father, John D. Bartels, MD, in private obstetrics and gynecology practice. They grew the practice to eventually include eight physicians. Dr. Bartels has been in private practice for 37 years and has delivered thousands of babies. He has sat on multiple committees at the Medical Society of the State of New York and represented western New York as Eighth District councilor for multiple terms and currently serves as Eighth District president.

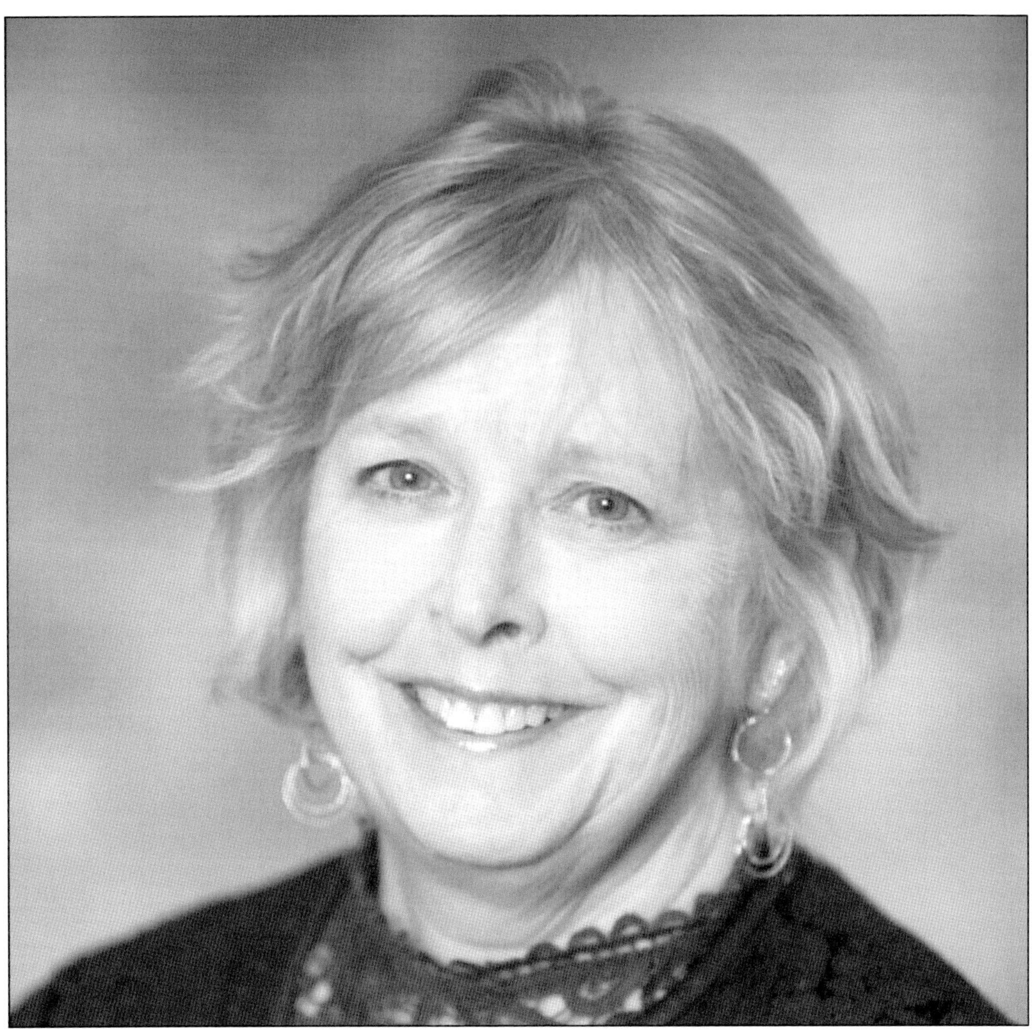

Dr. Kathleen Grimm is one of few female presidents of the Medical Society of Erie County (2009) and is also a member of the board of directors at the society. In addition, she currently serves as clinical assistant professor of medicine at the SUNY Buffalo School of Medicine and Biomedical Sciences. Board certified in pediatrics, internal medicine, and hospice and palliative medicine, her prior roles have included a tenure at SUNY Buffalo's Division of Internal Medicine/Pediatrics, and as a practicing physician in the Adolescent Clinic of Women & Children's Hospital of Buffalo and Quaker Medical Associates. Previously, she was a registered nurse at Buffalo General Hospital and Lancaster General Hospital in Pennsylvania. She has received a number of awards for her leadership and practice, including the Canisius College Distinguished Alumni Award, the ECMC Foundation Chairman's Distinguished Service Award, and the Frederick B. Wilkes Pediatric Award. In addition, Dr. Grimm is a fellow of the American College of Physicians and the American Academy of Pediatrics.

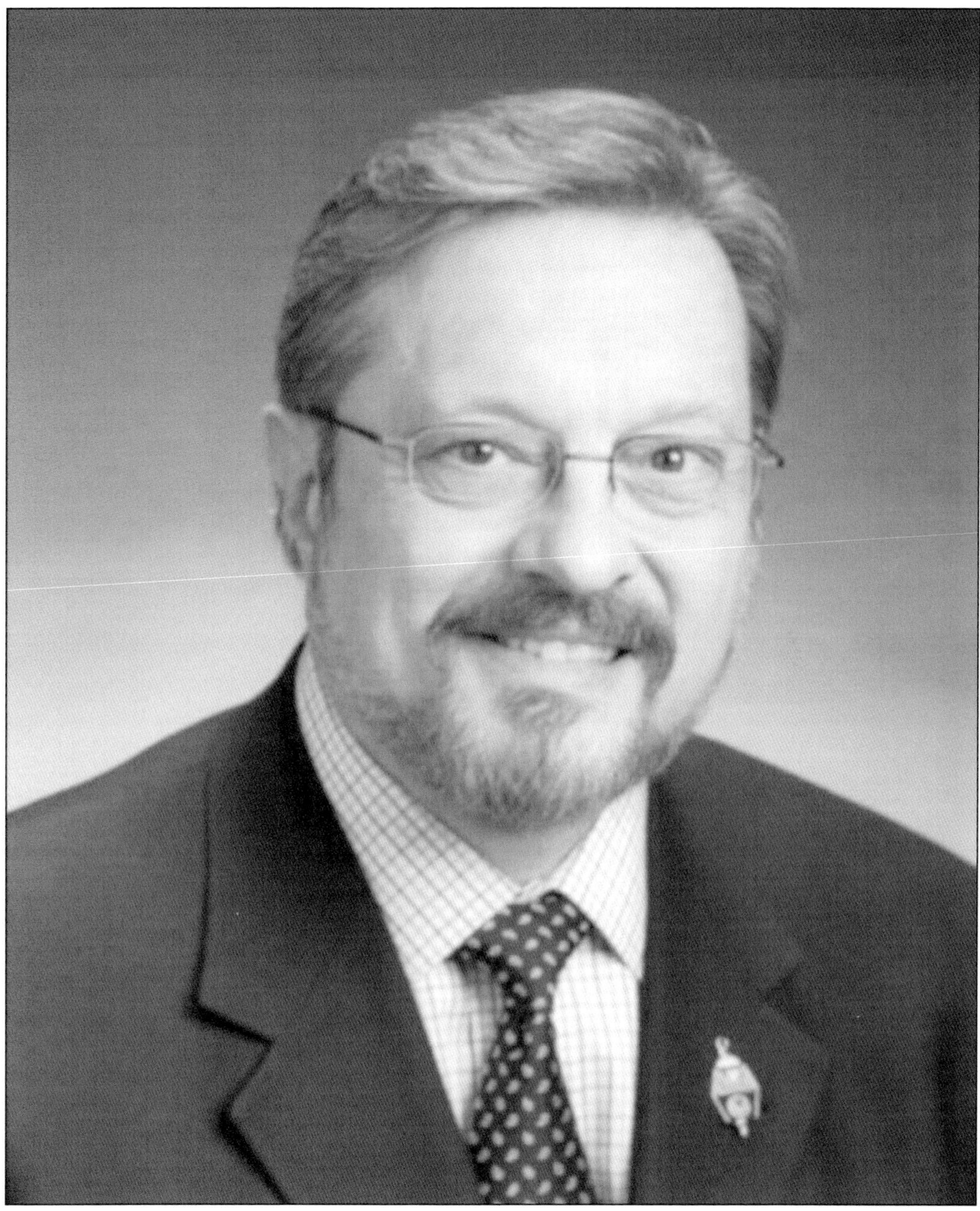

Mark J. Lema, MD, PhD, serves on the Medical Society 's executive board as past president (2011). He has chaired several of the society's committees and served as a delegate to MSSNY, served on various MSSNY committees, and was on the Eighth District's Advisory Council. Dr. Lema is professor of anesthesiology and oncology and chairman of the Department of Anesthesiology at Roswell Park Comprehensive Cancer Center. He is also a SUNY Distinguished Service Professor and chair of the SUNY Buffalo Department of Anesthesiology, Jacobs School of Medicine and Biomedical Sciences.

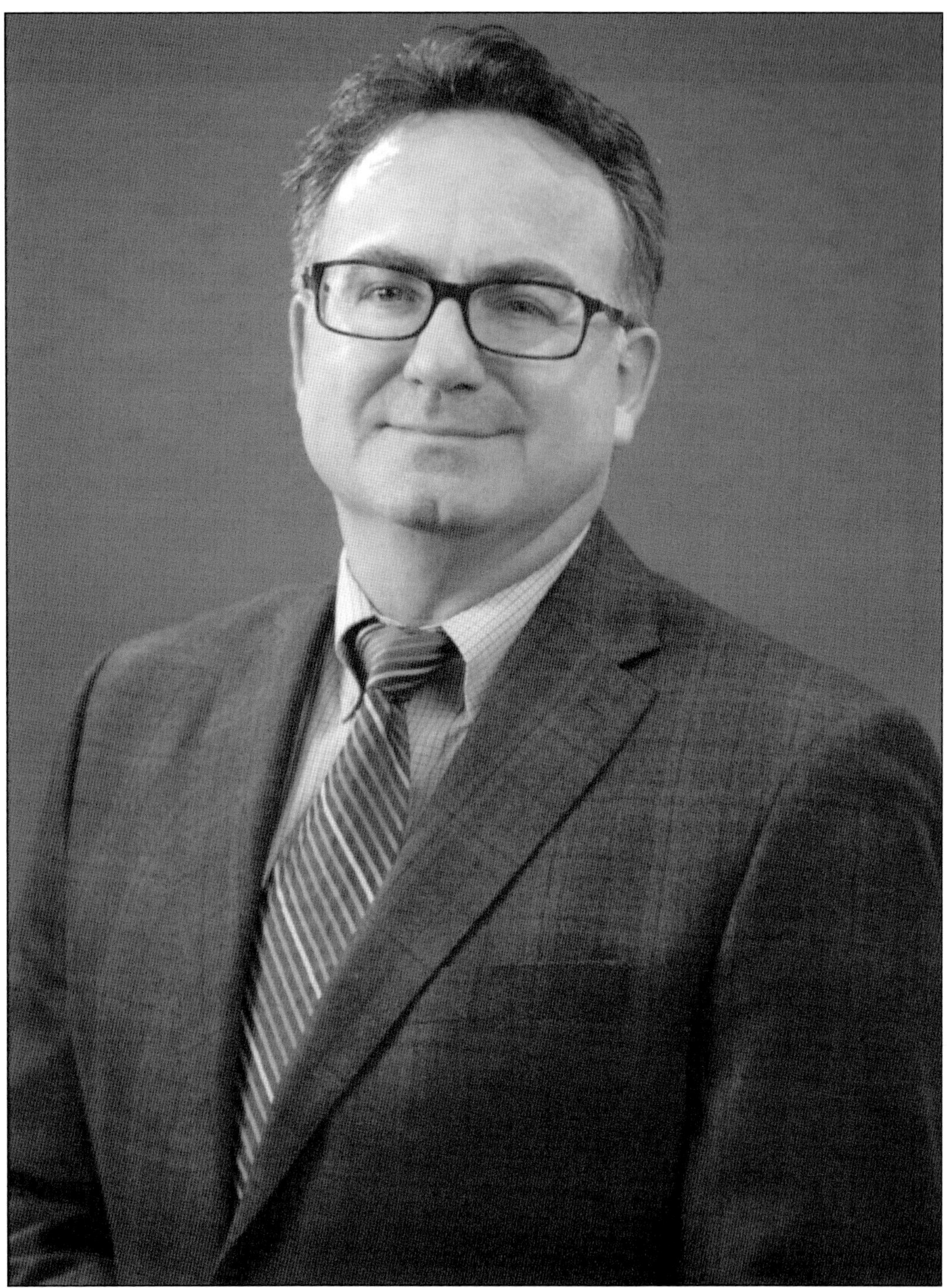

Raymond Paolini Jr., MD, received his medical degree from SUNY Buffalo in 1990 and has been practicing otolaryngology since he finished his postgraduate training at SUNY hospitals in Buffalo. He is a past president of the Medical Society (2012) and serves on the executive board. He has also served on several of the Medical Society's committees and is a Medical Society of the State of New York delegate.

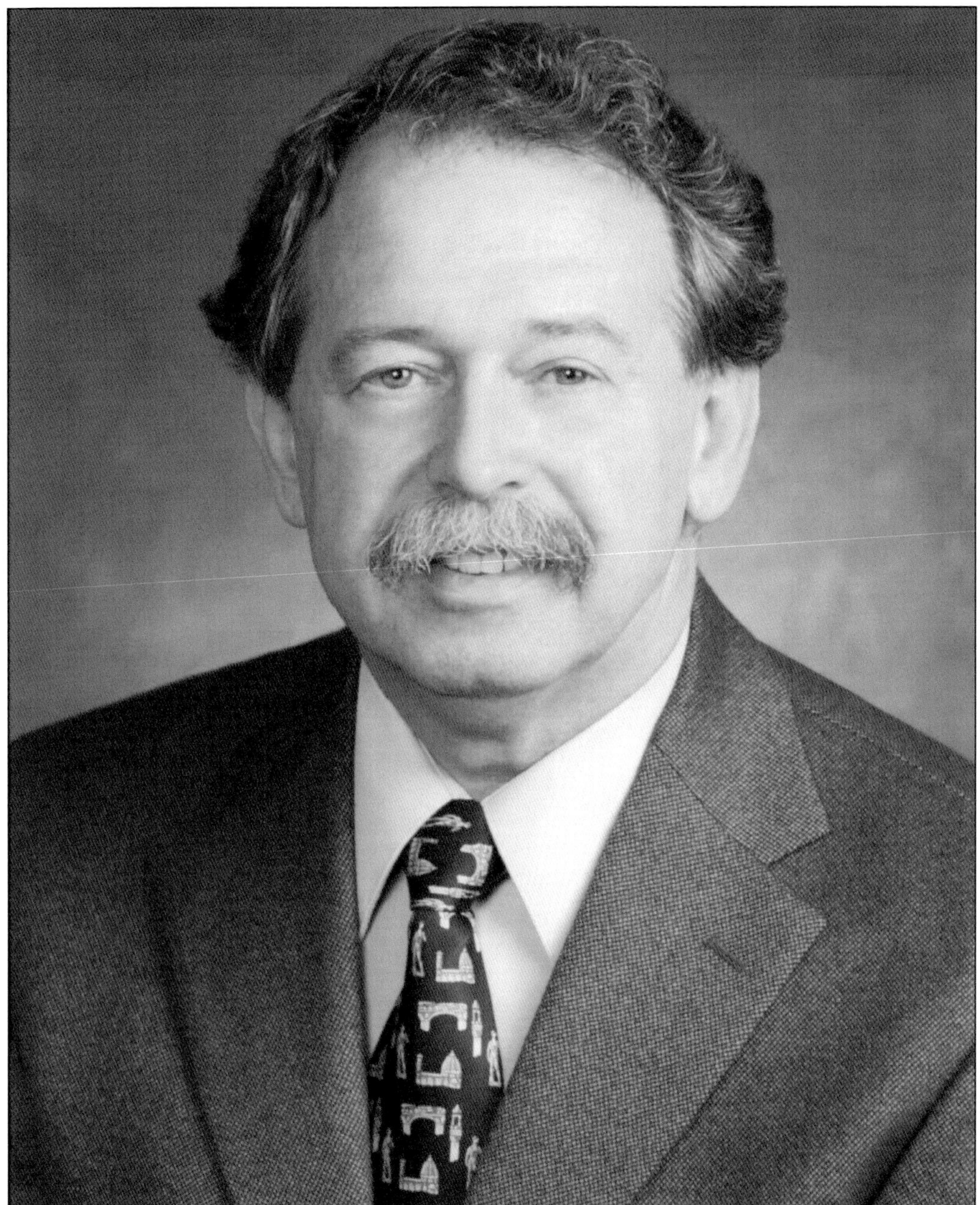

Dr. Timothy Gabryel is a board-certified general internist and a clinical professor of medicine, and was president of the Medical Society in 2016. He earned his undergraduate degree in 1972 and his doctor of medicine in 1976 from SUNY Buffalo. He completed his residency at Millard Fillmore Hospital in 1979. He was associate director of the SUNY Buffalo Internal Medicine Residency Program and was associate chair of medicine at Kaleida Health until 2000. He is currently the medical director at Mercy Hospital of Buffalo. He has sat on various committees at the county and state level and is an authority on resident and provider credentialing. In addition, he served on the MLMIC Insurance Company Board of Directors for many years. He continues to be an active primary care physician in West Seneca, New York.

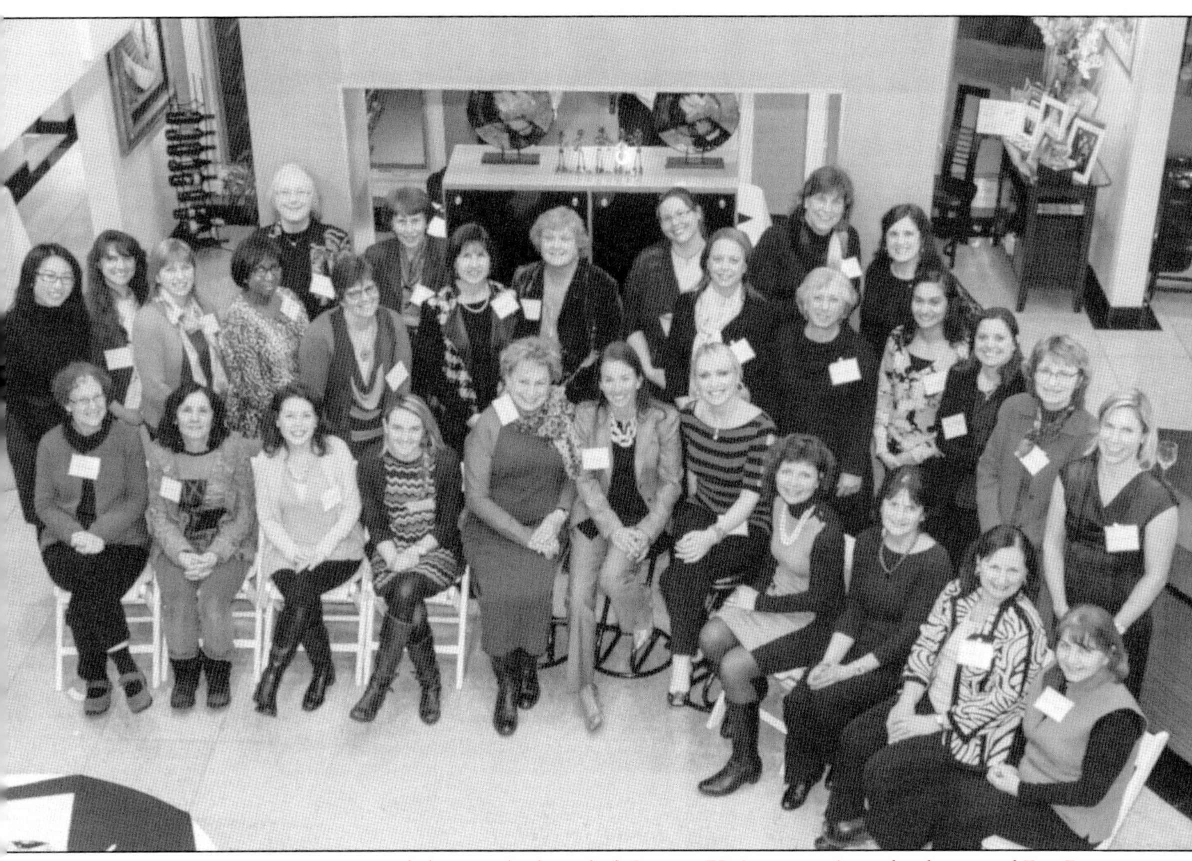

This was the first meeting of the newly founded DoctHERS in 2015 in the home of Dr. Rose Berkun. DoctHERS is a network of female physicians and scientists who address current issues in the medical fields in order to foster advancement, mentorship, and equal opportunities for women in medicine.

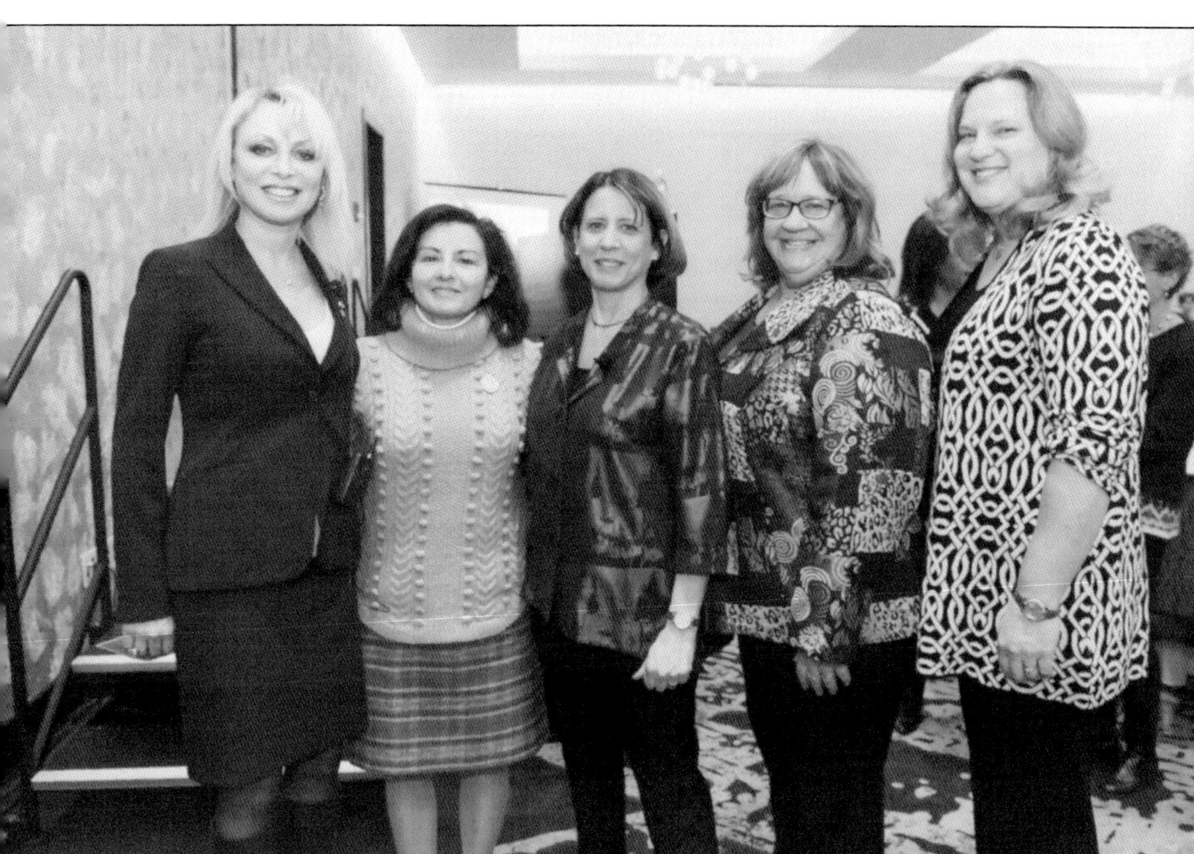

Pictured at the first annual DoctHERS Symposium in 2016 are, from left to right, Rose Berkun, MD; 2017 New York State Society of Anesthesiologists president Theresa Rorh-Hirchgraber, MD; 2016 American Medical Women's Association resident and keynote speaker Sara Laschiver; Roberta Gebhard, MD; and 2019 American Medical Women's Association president Stacey Watt, MD, the program director of anesthesiology at SUNY Buffalo.

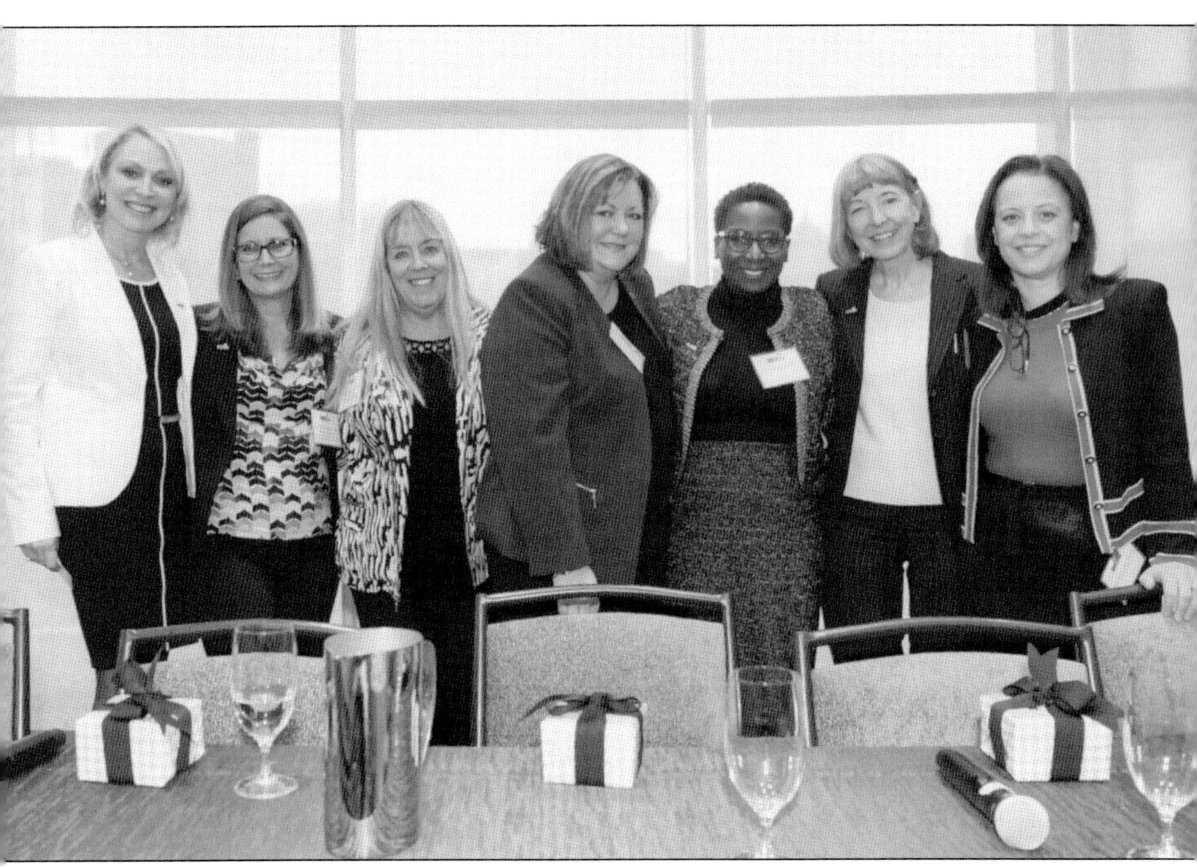

Shown here are female physician leaders at the 2018 DoctHERS Symposium. From left to right are Rose Berkun, MD, FASA; Lisa Jane Jacobsen, MD, MPH, MSHPEd, current president and CEO of Catholic Medical Partners; Margaret Paroski, MD; Jean Wactawski-Wende, PhD; Emmekunla Nylander, MD; Candace Johnson, PhD; and Helen Cappuccino, MD.

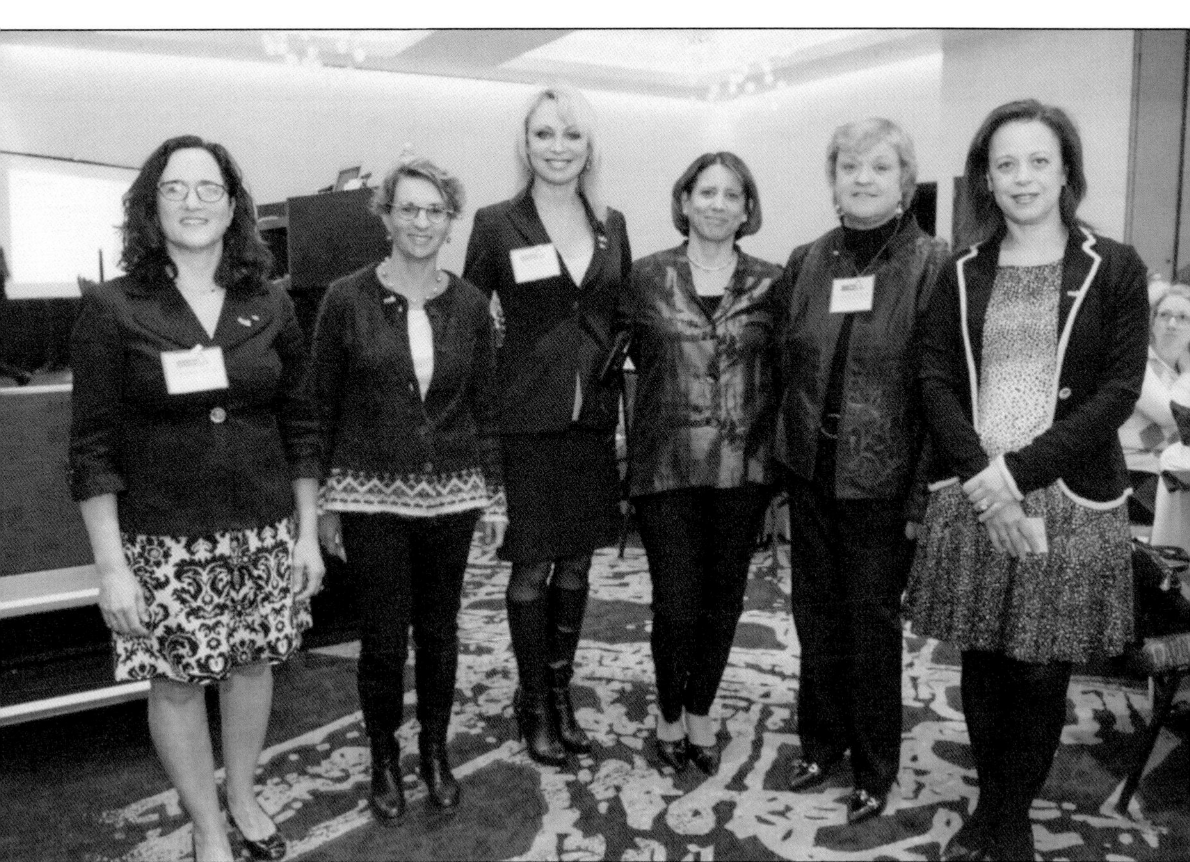

Attending the first annual DoctHERS Symposium in 2016 are, from left to right, Iris Danzinger, MD, founder and president of Amherst Southgate ENT; Erie County health commissioner Gale Burstein, MD, MPH; anesthesiologist and Medical Society of Erie County vice president Rose Berkun; Sara Laschiver; Dr. Nancy Nielsen, the first female president of the Medical Society and past president of the American Medical Association; and Helen Cappuccino, MD.

Willie Underwood III, MD, MSc, MPH, is a board-certified urologist with nearly 20 years of overall urologic surgery experience, including more than 10 years dedicated to robotic urologic surgery. He was elected to the American Medical Association Board of Trustees in June 2019. An expert in health care disparities and health care policy, Dr. Underwood has served on several national and regional health care policy committees, including as a board member of HealthNow, as a board member and medical advisor to the Love Canal Medical Fund Inc., as a past president of the Medical Society of Erie County, as a member of the AMA and National Medical Association Commission to End Health Care Disparities, and as a member of the Accreditation Council for Graduate Medical Education Urology Residency Review Committee. Dr. Underwood has also chaired the AMA Council on Legislation, the Medical Society of Erie County Legislative Affairs Committee, the Medical Society of the State of New York Quality Improvement and Patient Safety Committee, and the HealthNow Health Care Services and Quality Initiative Committee. He served as Medical Society president in 2017.

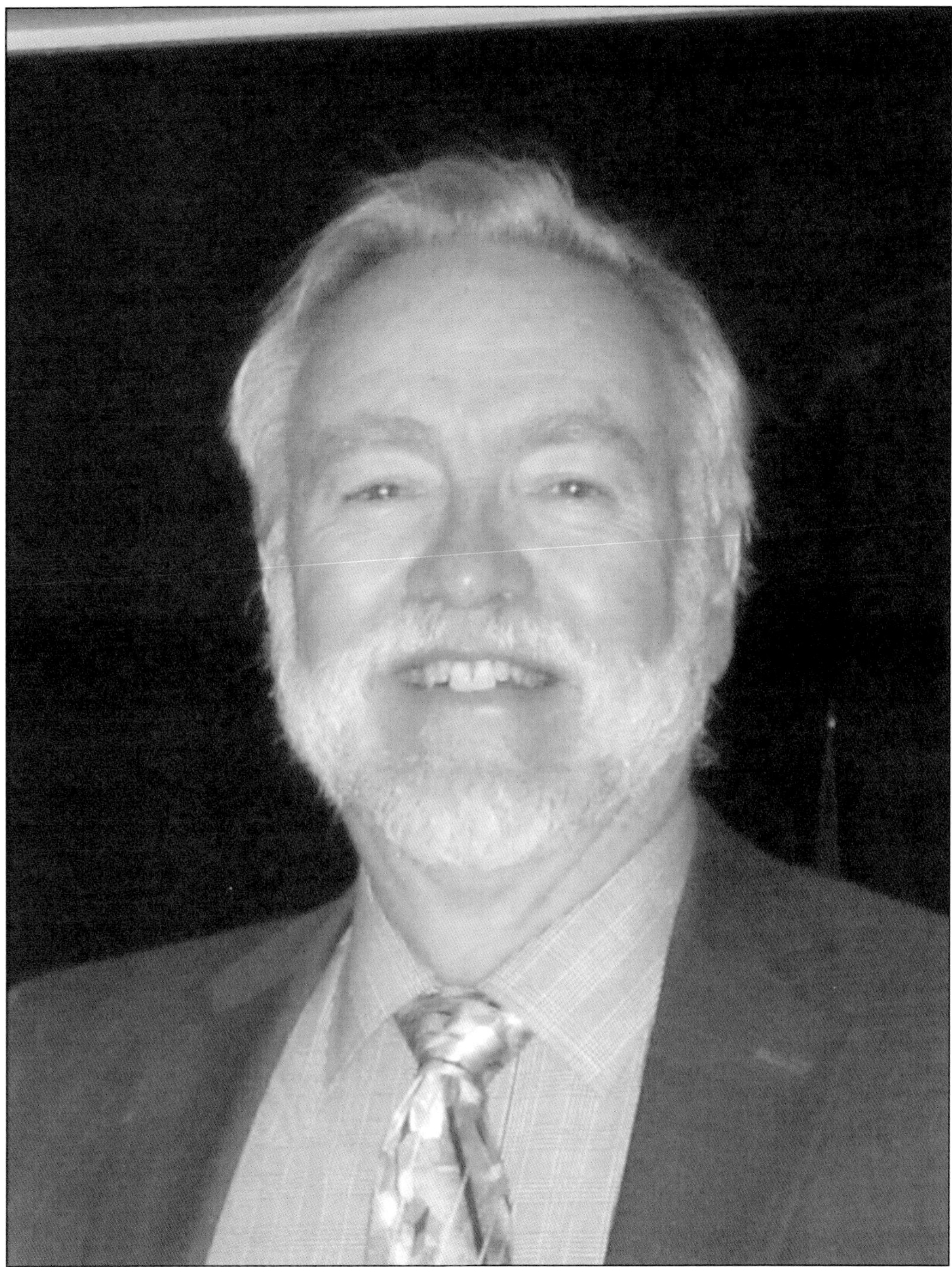

John Gillespie, MD, MMM, was president of the Medical Society of Erie County in 2018. He completed his undergraduate degree at Notre Dame University and obtained his medical degree from Boston University. A renowned cardiologist, he served as chief medical officer of Independent Health from 2007 to 2009 and chief medical officer of Palladian Health from 2010 to 2016. He also served as chief of cardiology at Highland Hospital in Rochester, New York, and sat as a member of the faculty of the University of Rochester and the University at Buffalo.

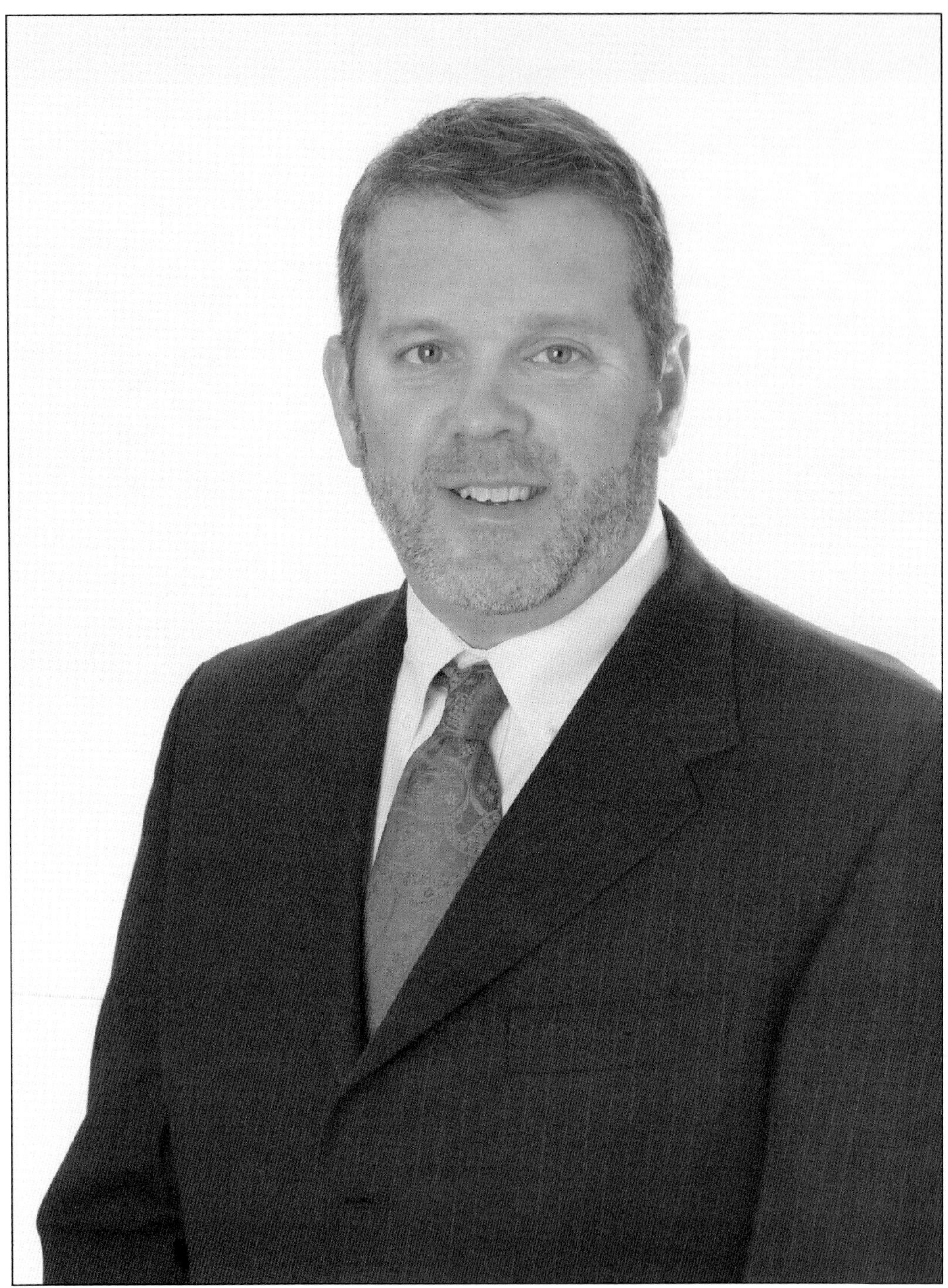

Kenneth H. Eckhert III, MD, was the third Medical Society president in his family when he served in 2019–2020. As a clinical assistant professor of surgery at the University at Buffalo School of Medicine, Dr. Eckhert teaches and mentors medical students and serves on several committees within regional hospitals in the community. Dr. Eckhert has been actively involved with Friends of Good Samaritan and served as a board member for the annual expeditions to Haiti.

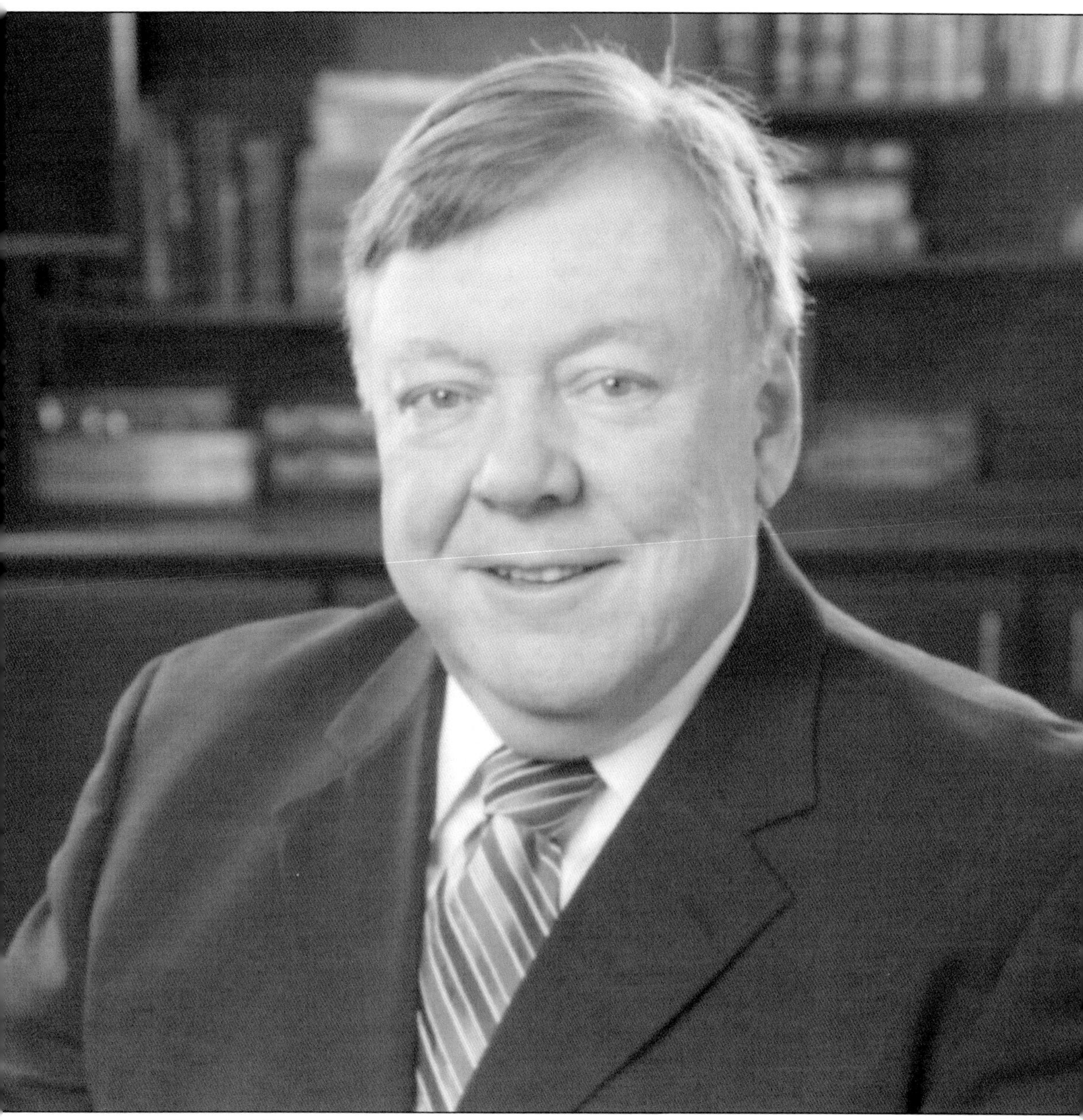

Stanley J. Pietrak, MD, is the current president of the Medical Society of Erie County (2020–2021). Dr. Pietrak had a noteworthy and heroic start to his career while stationed in Bosnia in 1996 with the US Army Reserves. Dr. Pietrak set up a gastrointestinal unit at the 65th Combat Support Hospital, performing procedures on patients ranging from liver disease to Crohn's disease. Currently, Dr. Pietrak practices at Gastroenterology Associates LLP in Amherst, New York.

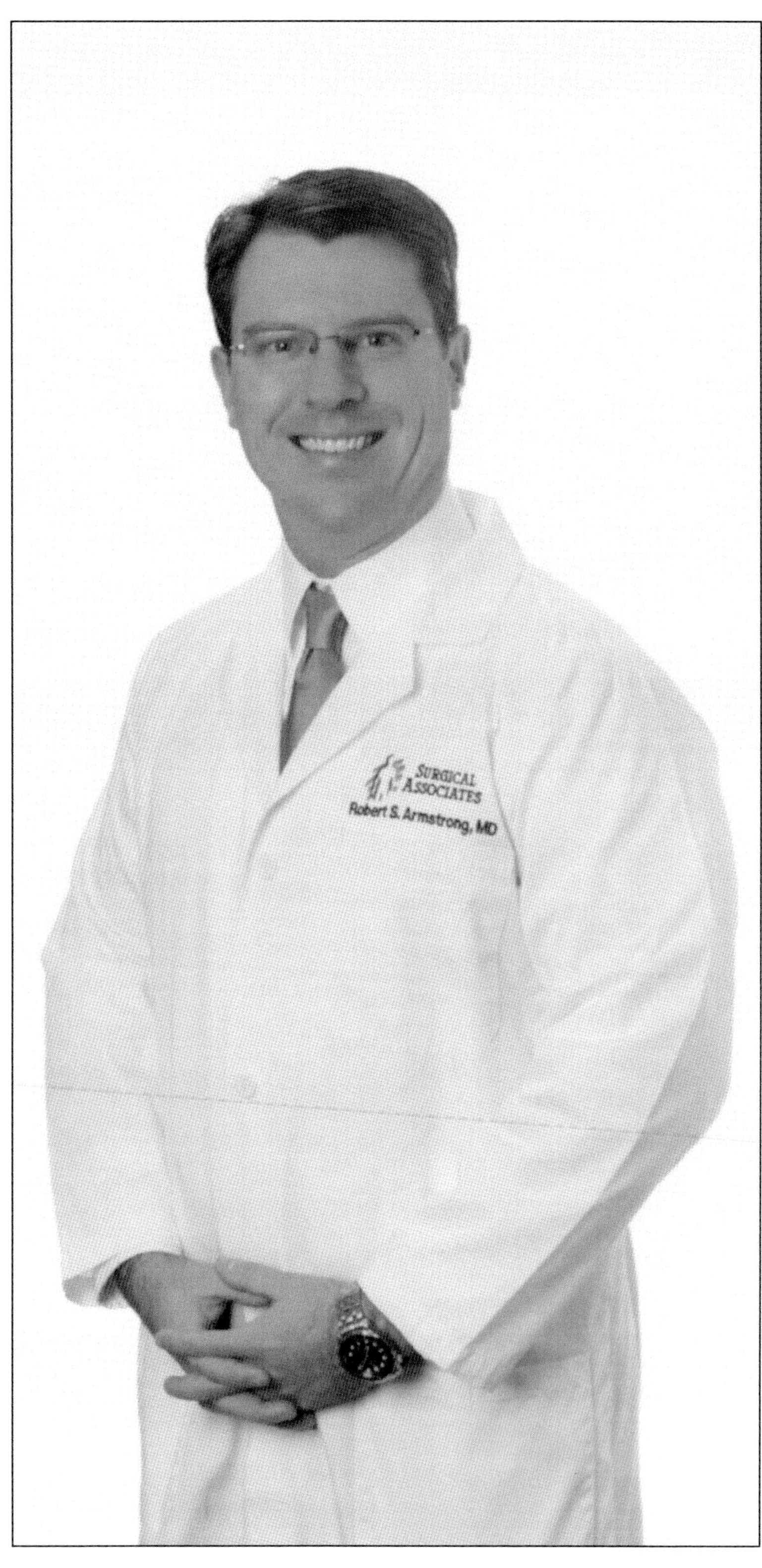

Robert S. Armstrong, MD, stands as the incoming 200th president of the Medical Society of Erie County. Dr. Armstrong graduated cum laude from the University of Dayton and completed his medical degree from the Boonshoft School of Medicine at Wright State University. He is a member the Medical Society of the State of New York, the Buffalo Surgical Society, the American Hernia Society, the American Medical Association, and the American College of Surgeons. Today, he practices at Surgical Associates of Western New York, PC.

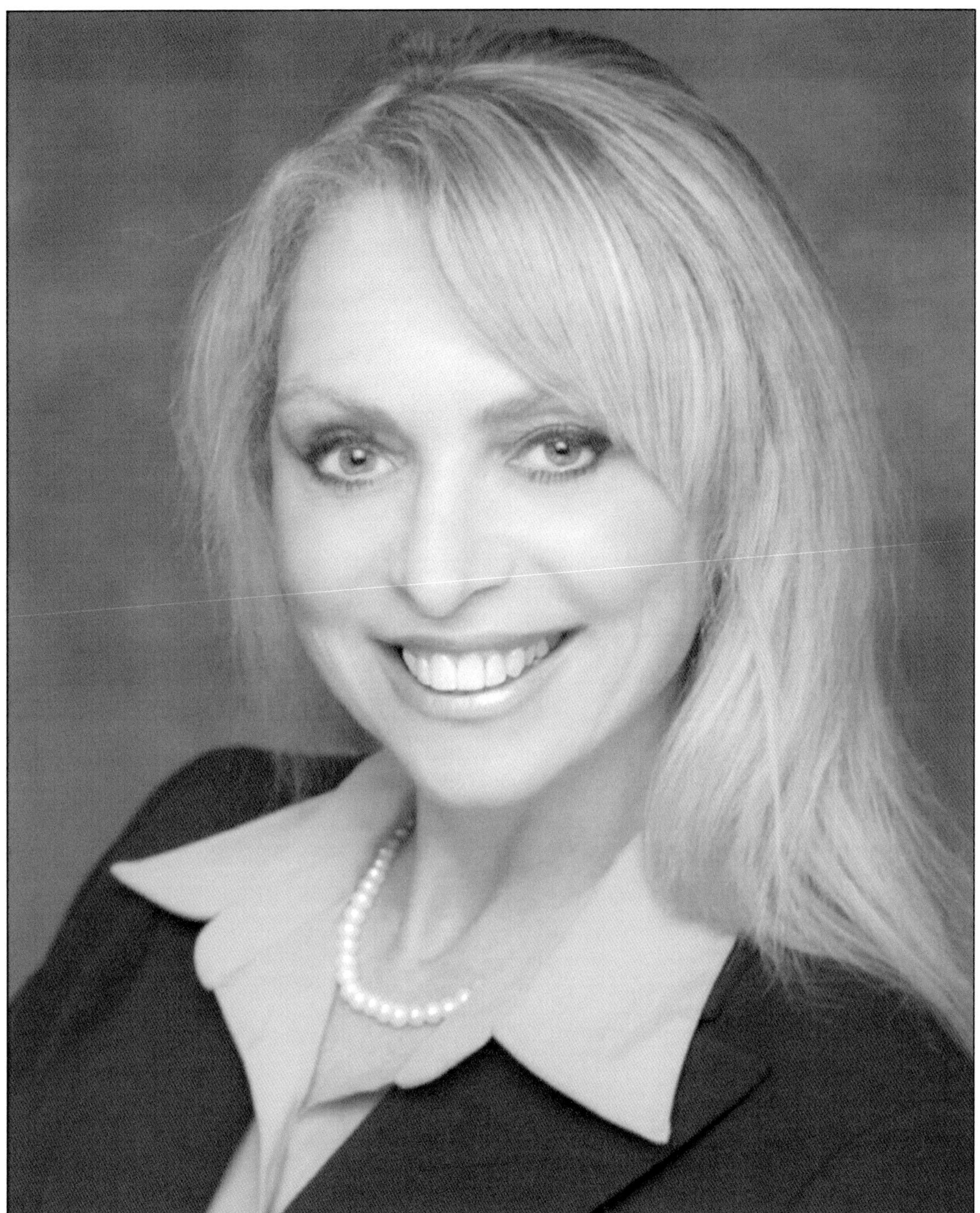

Rose Berkun, MD, is the current vice president of the Medical Society of Erie County (2020–2021) and past president of NYSSA. Dr. Berkun graduated cum laude from SUNY Buffalo in 1987, completed her medical degree at the SUNY Buffalo School of Medicine in 1992, and completed her anesthesia residency at SUNY Buffalo. Dr. Berkun's achievements include clinical associate professor seat at the SUNY Buffalo School of Medicine; medical director of anesthesia services at Aesthetic Associates Center; and founder of DoctHERS, a networking group for female physicians and scientists. She has also served on numerous committees at the local, state, and national level. In 2022, Dr. Berkun will serve as only the seventh female president in the Medical Society of Erie County's 200-year history.

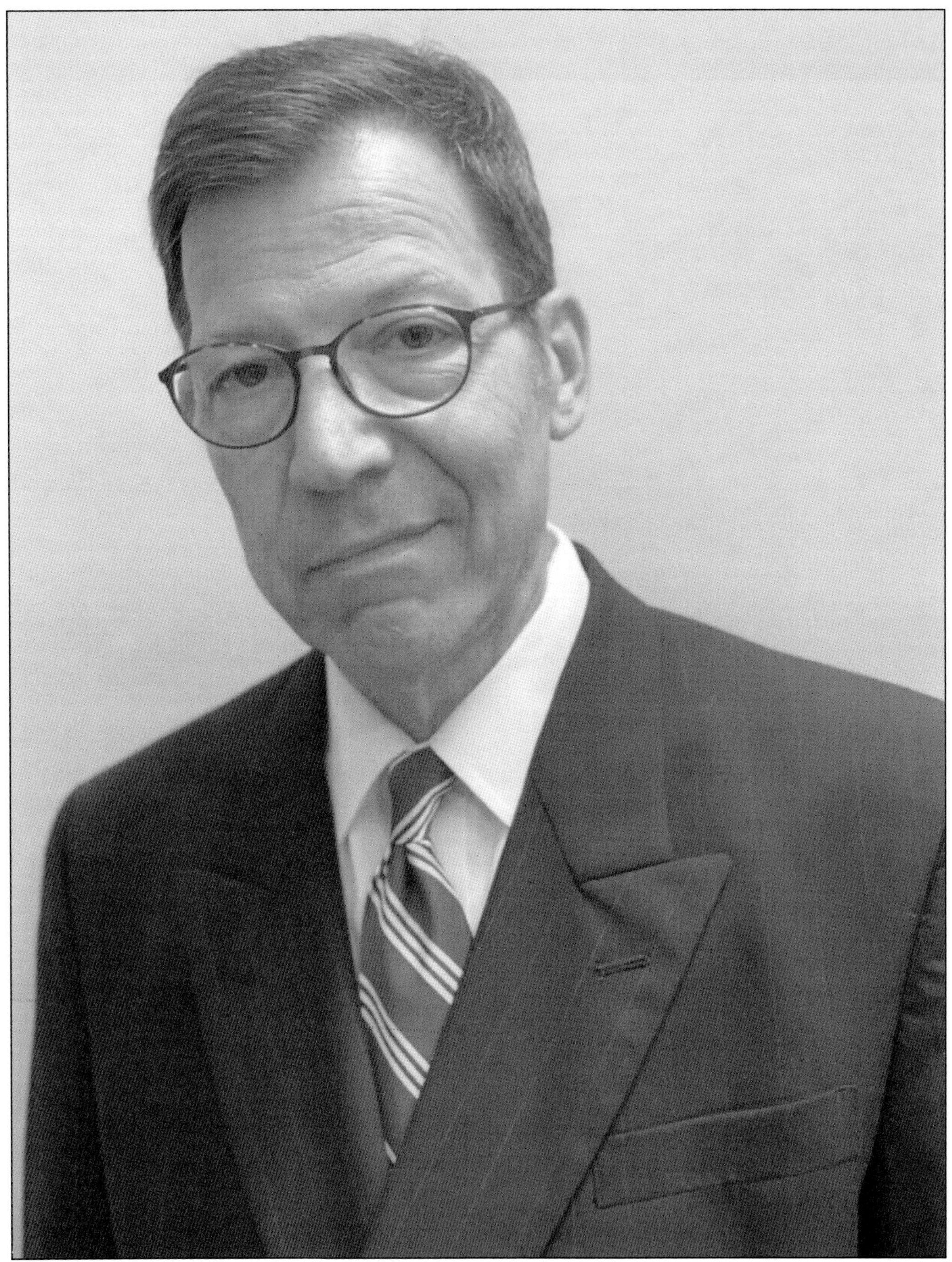

Michael Licata, DDS, MD, received his undergraduate, dental, and medical degrees from SUNY Buffalo. He did his internship and residency at SUNY Buffalo and practices with the same radiology group (Southtowns Radiology) that he joined 27 years ago. Dr. Licata is chair of the Medical Society of Erie County's Ethics Committee, which he has served on for the past 11 years.

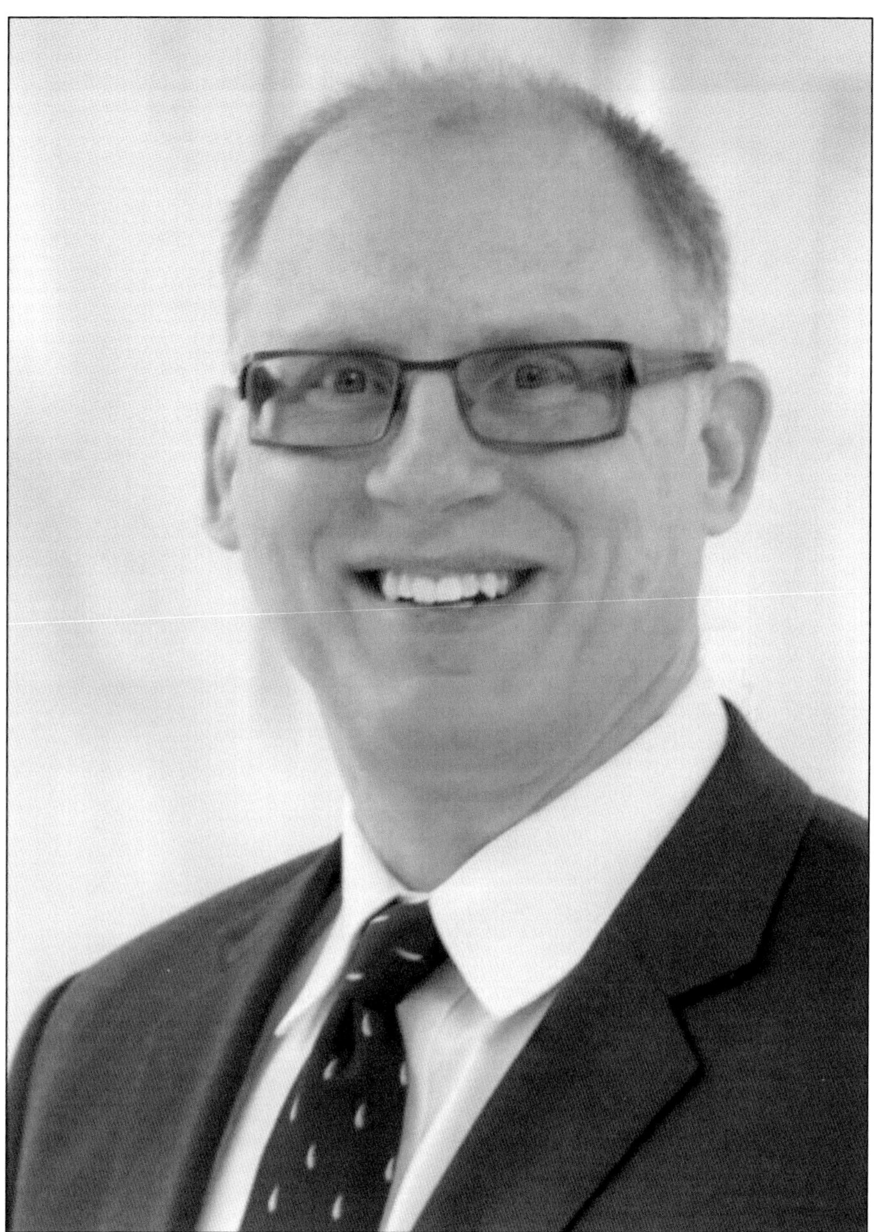

Dr. Todd Demmy, MD, received his undergraduate degree from Penn State University and his medical degree from Jefferson Medical College in 1983. Dr. Demmy is board certified by the American Board of Thoracic Surgery and has served in a number of leadership capacities as assistant professor of surgery, codirector of cardiac transplantation, chief of thoracic oncology from 1994 to 2002, and chair of the Medical Society of Erie County's Medical Services Committee. Dr. Demmy has achieved a very high reliability in performing minimally invasive operations for the most complex tumors, and by communicating these enabling techniques to other surgeons by annotated video productions, he has received national and international recognition. He has written articles in peer-reviewed journals as well as book chapters and presents regularly at national and international professional meetings. Dr. Demmy currently practices as a thoracic surgeon at Roswell Park Comprehensive Cancer Center in Buffalo, New York.

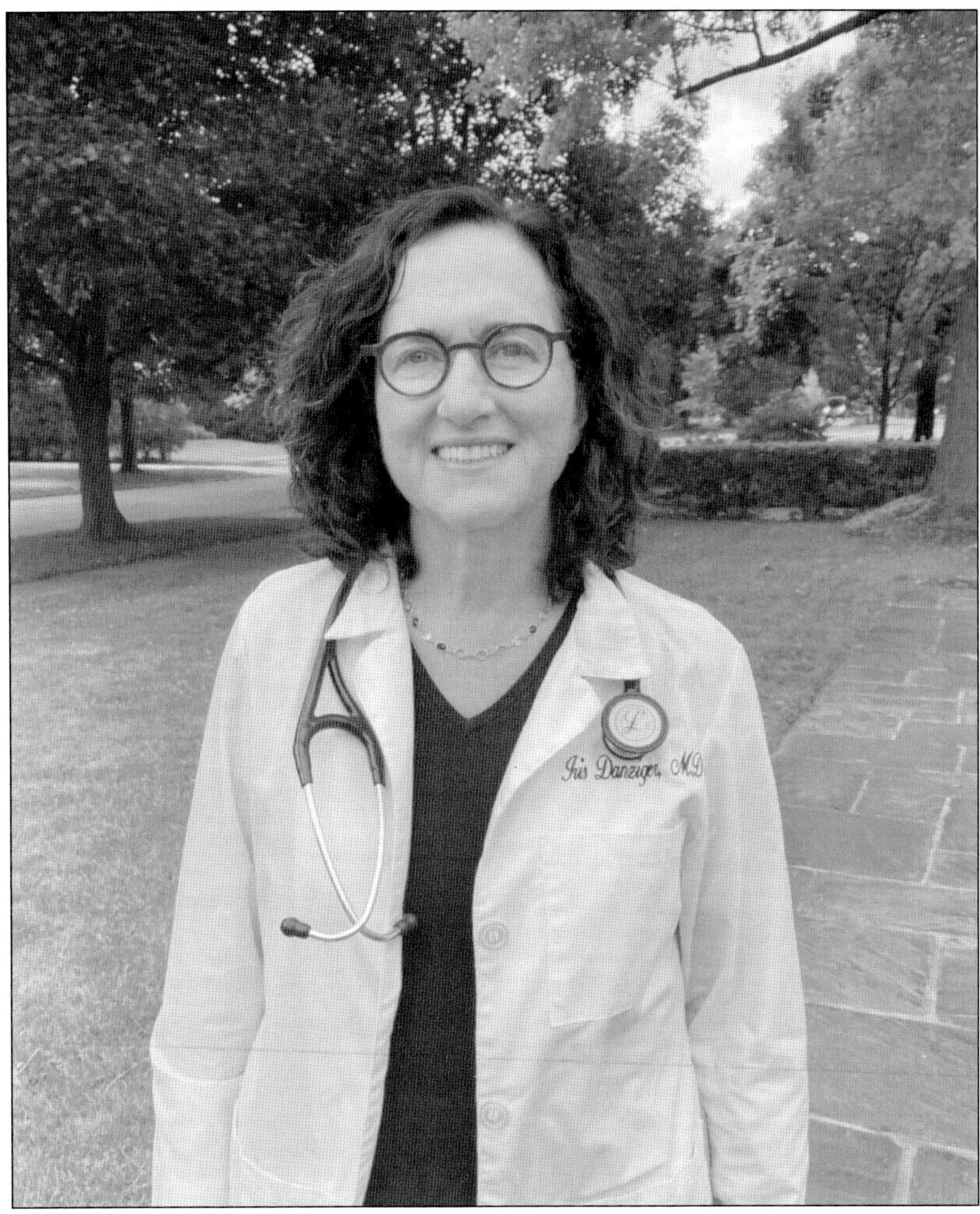

Board certified in otolaryngology, Iris Danziger, MD, is the current chair of the New Physicians in Practice Committee and board member of the Medical Society. Dr. Danziger graduated from SUNY Buffalo School of Medicine and Biomedical Sciences and also completed her residency in otolaryngology and head and neck surgery at SUNY Buffalo. Dr. Danziger is an assistant clinical professor at the Jacobs School of Medicine and Biomedical Sciences. She has received numerous awards and honors, including the Diversity and Inclusion Award from the Jacobs School of Medicine and Biomedical Sciences, Department of Otolaryngology in 2016, and the Norman Haber and Norman Stoller awards in 1986 and 1988, respectively. Dr. Danziger is the founder and president of Amherst Southgate ENT.

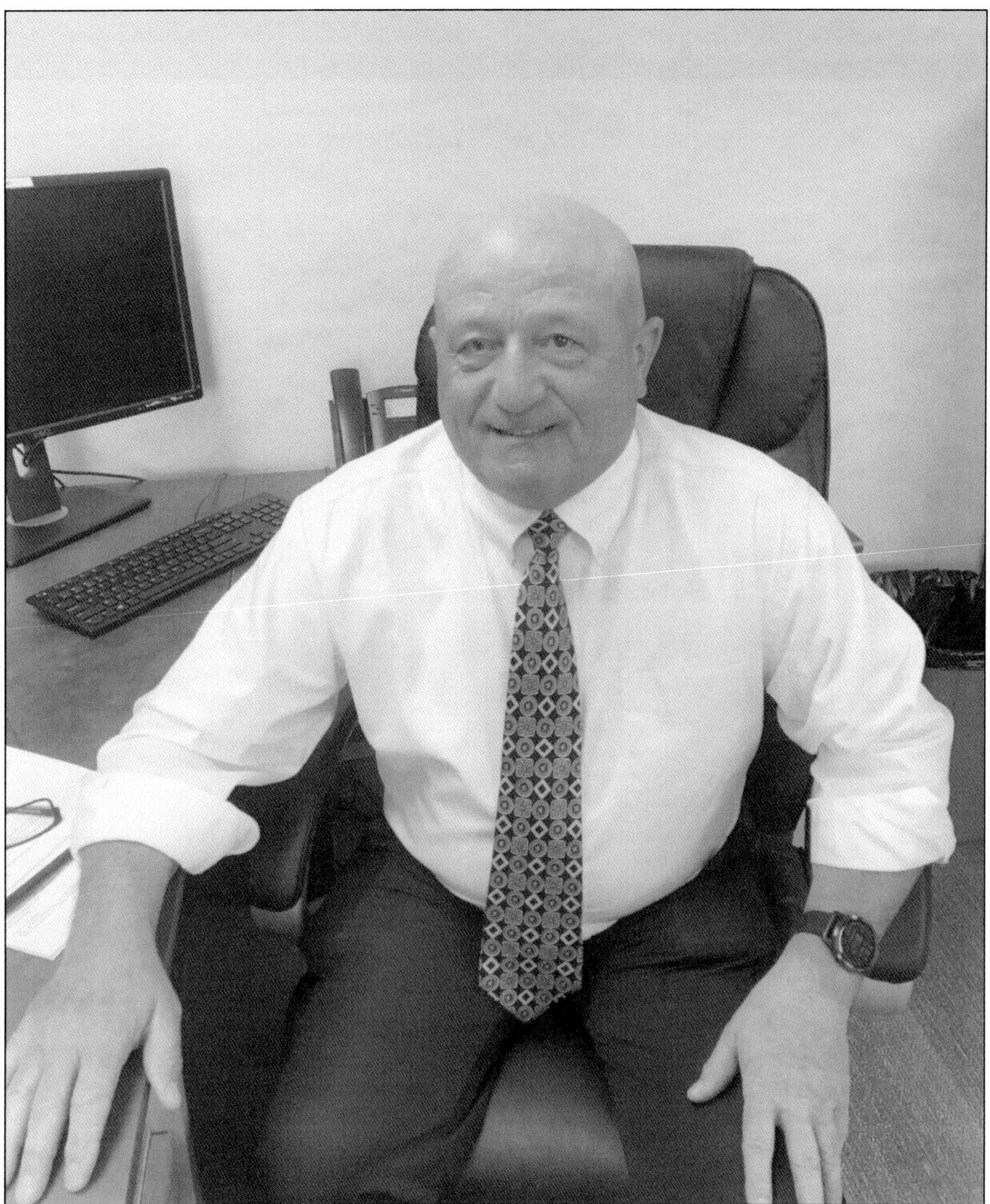

Gordon Tussing, DO, started his career as a pharmacist and obtained his doctor of osteopathic medicine in 1997 from Western University in Pomona, California. He completed his residency in internal medicine at Sisters of Charity Hospital in 2000. A group leader at Catholic IPA from 2005 to 2008, Dr. Tussing has created a longstanding leadership role in the medical community. His teaching appointments include SUNY School of Medicine and School of Pharmacy, Daemen Physician Assistant and Nurse Practitioner programs, and program director of the Osteopathic Internal Medicine Residency Program at Sisters of Charity Hospital. He sat on the Medical Society of Erie County's Health Law Committee from 2009 to 2013 and currently chairs the Practice Management Committee. Dr. Tussing remains a board member of the society and currently practices internal medicine in Snyder, New York.

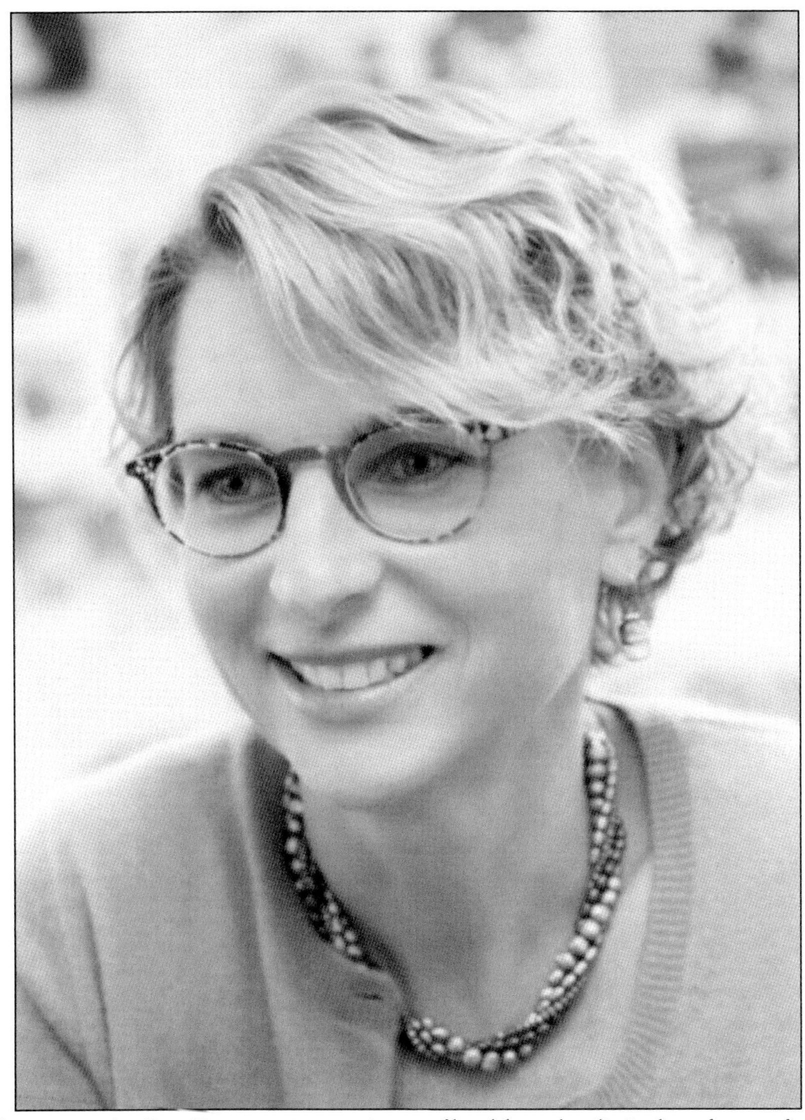

Dr. Gale Burstein is the Erie County commissioner of health and a clinical professor of pediatrics at the University at Buffalo Jacobs School of Medicine. She is currently leading Erie County's public health COVID-19 response. During the pandemic, Dr. Burstein continued working on strategies to expand substance abuse prevention and treatment services, prevent opioid related overdoses and deaths, expand access to sexual health care, increase hepatitis C virus testing and treatment, and decrease childhood lead toxicity. Dr. Burstein cochairs the Erie County Opioid Epidemic Task Force. She participates in writing national adolescent health care guidelines and has been published in many scientific peer review journals. Dr. Burstein earned her doctor of medicine from the SUNY Buffalo Jacobs School of Medicine; completed a pediatric residency at Case Western Reserve University in Cleveland, Ohio; received adolescent medicine fellowship training at the University of Maryland; and completed a Centers for Disease Control and Prevention sexually transmitted diseases prevention fellowship and a master's degree in public health from Johns Hopkins University in Baltimore, Maryland. As a CDC medical officer, she worked on adolescent sexually transmitted infection prevention programs, policy, and guidelines and directed the first national rapid HIV testing surveillance program.

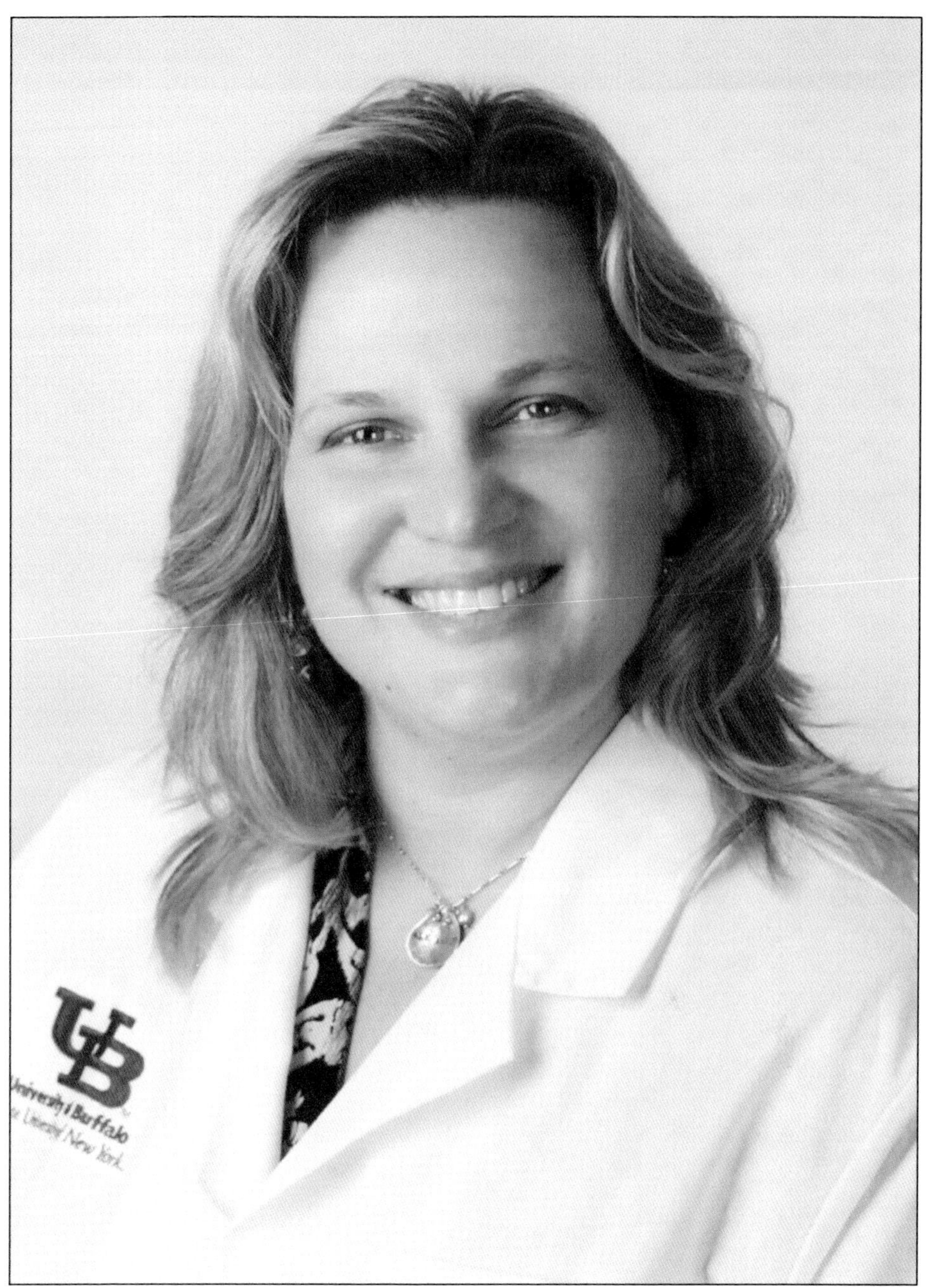

Dr. Stacey Watt is one of western New York's most highly acclaimed athletes, receiving a full athletic scholarship to the University of Florida for her number-one ranking in the discus event for all high school women in the nation. She went on to become a two-time NCAA All-American and US Olympic Festival medalist, representing the United States at the Pan-American Games. She has received numerous awards that celebrate her athletic achievements, which reside within many local, state, and regional athletic halls of fame. Her competitive nature and skills on the athletic field transitioned into the operating room, where she now leads her team at Kaleida Health and the University at Buffalo as both chief of service of the anesthesiology department and program director for the Anesthesiology Residency Program.

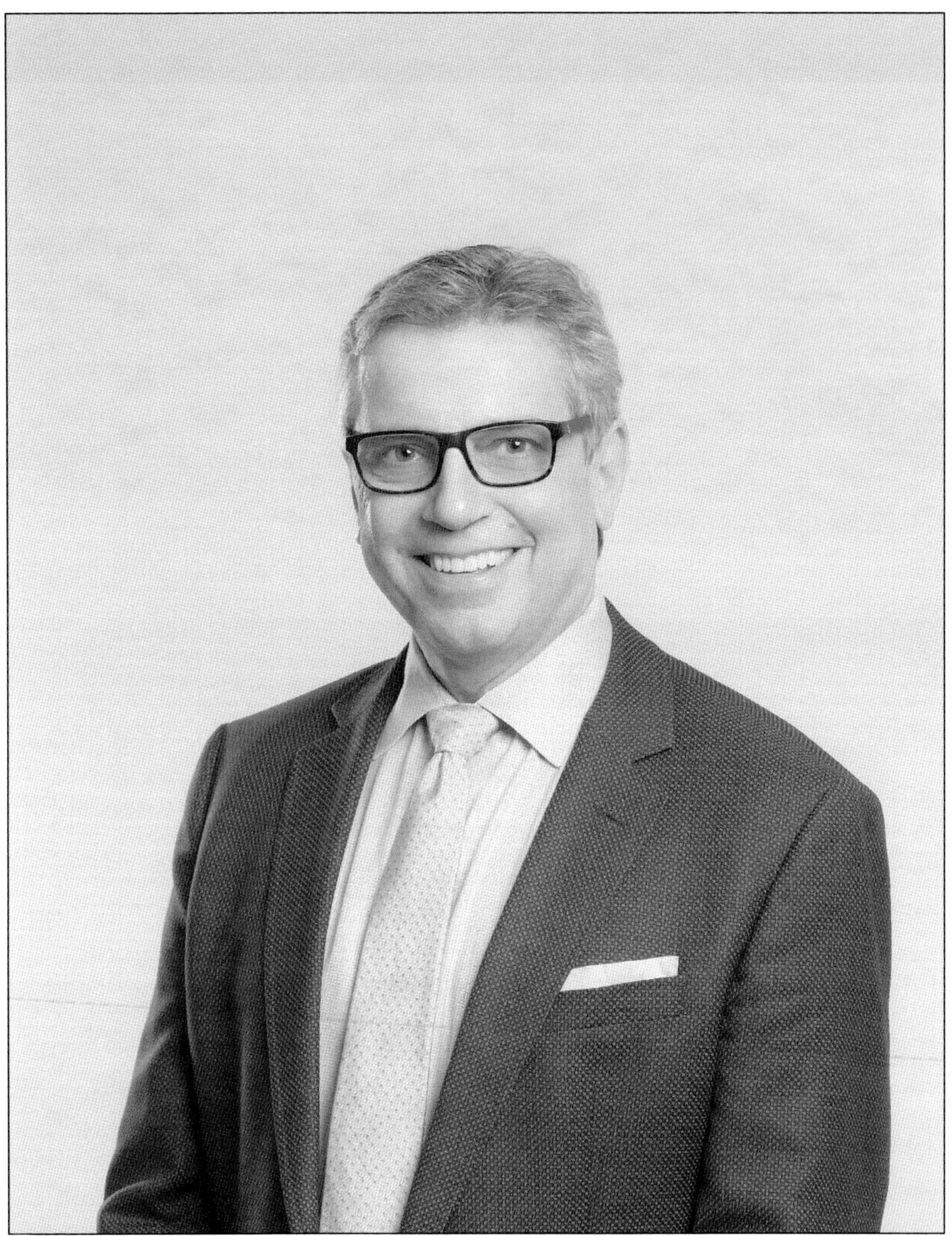

John Fudyma, MD, MPH, current treasurer of the Medical Society of Erie County and incoming vice president, serves as chief medical officer for Latus Medical Care. Dr. Fudyma has more than 40 years of experience in the medical field and most recently served as chief of division of general internal medicine for the University at Buffalo Jacobs School of Medicine and Biomedical Sciences. He received a master's degree in public health from Columbia University's Mailman School of Public Health.

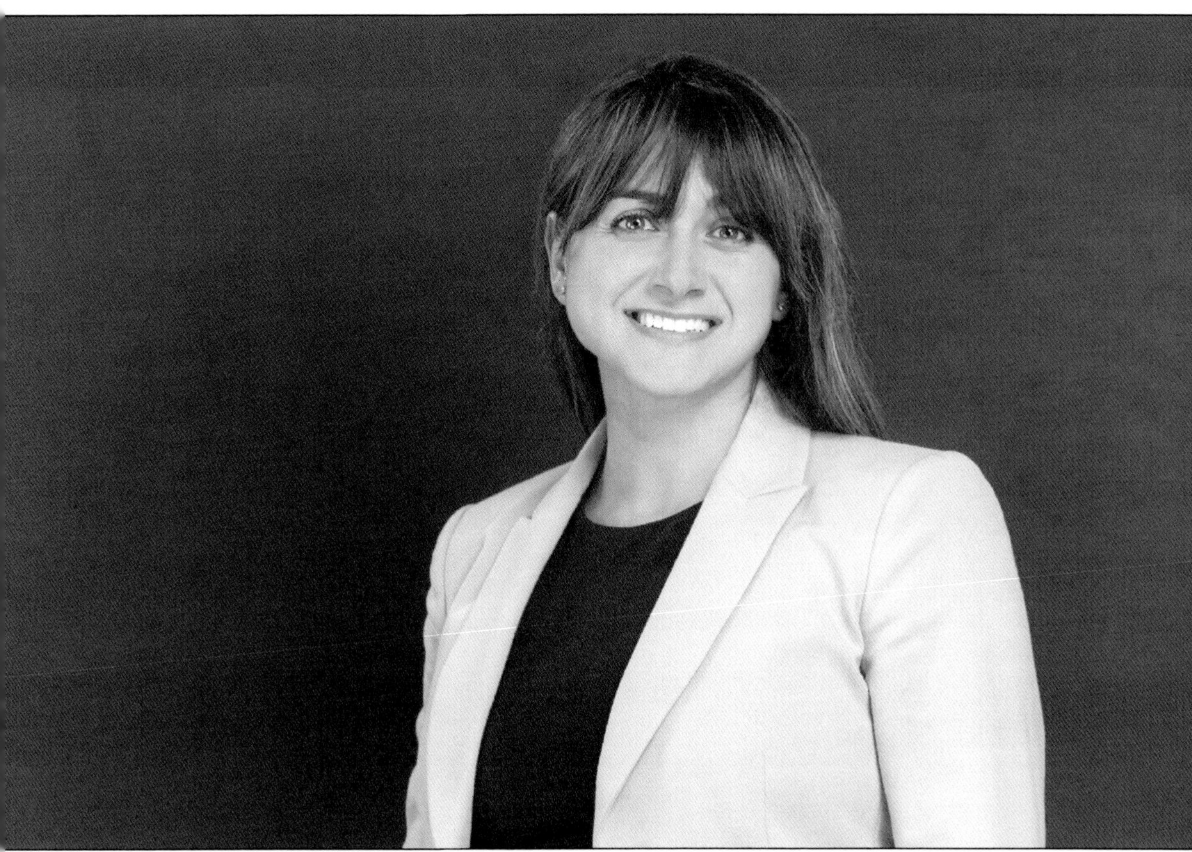

Aimana ElBahtity, Esq. joined the Medical Society of Erie County in July 2020 as executive director. She is an attorney who practiced insurance defense and health care law in New York and Chicago before moving to Washington, DC, where she worked at the US Department of Justice's 9/11 Victim Compensation Fund. She most recently directed the Risk Management Department and served as patient safety officer at a prominent Adventist Healthcare Medical Center in the DC metro area. She is a native of Buffalo, which is also home to her alma mater, the University at Buffalo School of Law.

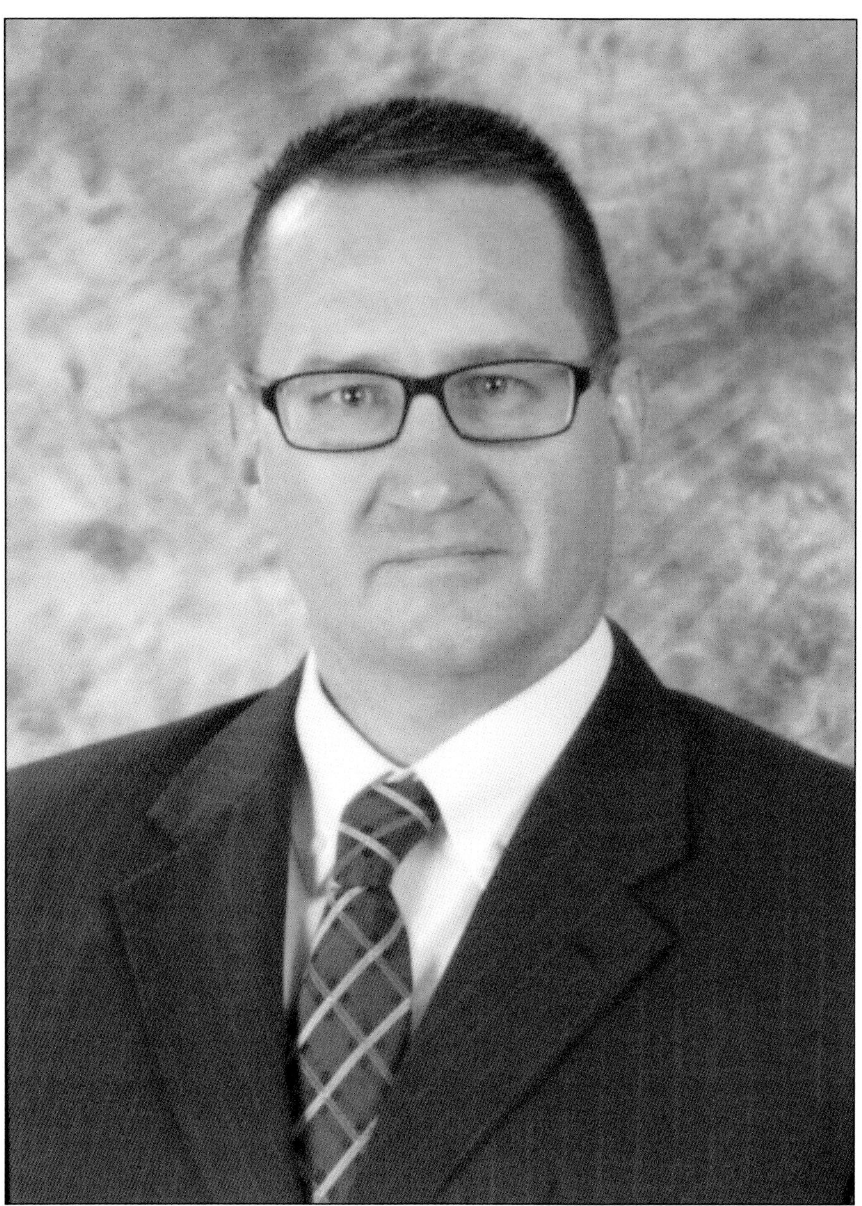

Dr. Mark R. Jajkowski is a native of Buffalo. Dr. Jajkowski completed his undergraduate studies at Canisius College. He then graduated from medical school at SUNY Buffalo, where he also completed a postgraduate residency in general surgery. Dr. Jajkowski then went on to complete fellowship training in cardiothoracic surgery at the University of Rochester. His practice focus is in the area of general thoracic surgery, particularly the treatment of lung cancer using minimally invasive techniques and robotic technology. Since 2018, he has been director of thoracic surgery for Catholic Health System and served as the first system-wide elected medical staff president from 2016 to 2018. Dr. Jajkowski has been a member of the Medical Society of Erie County and the Medical Society of the State of New York since 1998 and was selected as the Eighth District councilor to MSSNY in 2020. In addition, he has chaired the Legislative and Young Physician Committees for the Medical Society of Erie County. Dr. Jajkowski has also served as a delegate to the MSSNY House of Delegates since 2007, and as the 8th District councilor to MSSNY.

Past Presidents
Medical Society, County of Erie

1821	Cyrenius Chapin, M.D.	1872	William Ring, M.D.	1922	Dewitt H. Sherman, M.D.
1822	Cyrenius Chapin, M.D.	1873	Jabez Allen, M.D.	1923	Charles E. Abbott, M.D.
1823		1874	Thomas Lothrop, M.D.	1924	Julius H. Potter, M.D.
1824		1875	John Cronyn, M.D.	1925	Charles R. Borzilleri, M.D.
1825		1876	John Cronyn, M.D.	1926	Robert E. De Ceu, M.D.
1826		1877	Henry Lapp, M.D.	1927	W. Warren Britt, M.D.
1827		1878	Edward Storck, M.D.	1928	Francis M. O'Gorman, M.D.
1828	Bela H. Colegrove, M.D.	1879	Sylvester F. Mixer, M.D.	1929	Baldwin Mann, M.D.
1829	Bela H. Colegrove, M.D.	1880	F. F. Hoyer, M.D.	1930	William T. Getman, M.D.
1830	John E. Marshall, M.D.	1881	John Hauenstein, M.D.	1931	Marshall Clinton, M.D.
1831		1882	T. M. Johnson, M.D.	1932	Edward L. Villiaume, M.D.
1832		1883	S. E. S. H. Nott, M.D.	1933	Edward A. Sharp, M.D.
1833	Moses Bristol, M.D.	1884	Joseph C. Greene, M.D.	1934	James H. Borrell, M.D.
1834	Carlos Emmons, M.D.	1885	Judson B. Andrews, M.D.	1935	Herbert H. Bauckus, M.D.
1835	Alden S. Sprague, M.D.	1886	E. T. Dorland, M.D.	1936	Milton G. Potter, M.D.
1836	H. H. Bissell, M.D.	1887	O. C. Strong, M.D.	1937	John T. Donovan, M.D.
1837	James E. Hawley, M.D.	1888	J. D. Hill, M.D.	1938	Harry C. Guess, M.D.
1838	Moses Bristol, M.D.	1889	Rollin L. Banta, M.D.	1939	Carlton E. Wertz, M.D.
1839	Josiah Trowbridge, M.D.	1890	G. W. McPherson, M.D.	1940	Herbert E. Wells, M.D.
1840	Erastus Wallis, M.D.	1891	E. C. W. O'Brien, M.D.	1941	Nelson W. Strohm, M.D.
1841	Gordon F. Pratt, M.D.	1892	William Warren Potter, M.D.	1942	Harvey P. Hoffman, M.D.
1842	Josiah Barnes, M.D.	1893	John Parmenter, M.D.	1943	Harold F. Brown, M.D.
1843	J. B. Pride, M.D.	1894	William H. Gail, M.D.	1944	John D. Naples, M.D.
1844	William K. Scott, M.D.	1895	F. W. Bartlett, M.D.	1945	A. H. Aaron, M.D.
1845	Orlando Wakelee, M.D.	1896	J. G. Thompson, M.D.	1946	Porter A. Steele, M.D.
1846	Francis L. Harris, M.D.	1897	Henry R. Hopkins, M.D.	1947	Arthur F. Glaeser, M.D.
1847	Isaac Parsell, M.D.	1898	Lucien C. Howe, M.D.	1948	E. Dean Babbage, M.D.
1848	Charles H. Austin, M.D.	1899	John B. Coakley, M.D.	1949	Roy L. Scott, M.D.
1849	Erastus Wallis, M.D.	1900	E. H. Ballou, M.D.	1950	Stephen A. Graczyk, M.D.
1850	Charles H. Wilcox, M.D.	1901	William C. Phelps, M.D.	1951	Elmer T. McGroder, M.D.
1851	Alden S. Sprague, M.D.	1902	Walden M. Ward, M.D.	1952	Samuel Sanes, M.D.
1852	Lewis J. Ham, M.D.	1903	Ernest Wende, M.D.	1953	William J. Orr, M.D.
1853	Phineas H. Strong, M.D.	1904	William E. Krauss, M.D.	1954	Antonio F. Bellanca, M.D.
1854	John G. House, M.D.	1905	John D. McPherson, M.D.	1955	Walter Scott Walls, M.D.
1855	James P. White, M.D.	1906	A. H. Briggs, M.D.	1956	Matthew J. Callanan, M.D.
1856	William Van Pelt, M.D.	1907	A. H. Briggs, M.D.	1957	Matthew L. Carden, M.D.
1857	Frank H. Hamilton, M.D.	1908	Edward Clark, M.D.	1958	Max Cheplove, M.D.
1858	Austin Flint, M.D.	1909	Charles A. Wall, M.D.	1959	Thomas S. Bumbalo, M.D.
1859	L. P. Dayton, M.D.	1910	Grover W. Wende, M.D.	1960	Kenneth H. Eckhert, M.D.
1860	William Treat, M.D.	1911	Daniel V. McClure, M.D.	1961	Eugene J. Hanavan, M.D.
1861	Sandford Eastman, M.D.	1912	Thomas H. McKee, M.D.	1962	Clarence A. Straubinger, M.D.
1862	James B. Samo, M.D.	1913	J. F. Whitwell, M.D.	1963	Walter T. Zimdahl, M.D.
1863	Charles Winne, M.D.	1914	John V. Woodruff, M.D.	1964	Francis W. O'Donnell, M.D.
1864	Cornelius C. Wyckoff, M.D.	1915	Arthur W. Hurd, M.D.	1965	Herbert E. Joyce, M.D.
1865	Charles C. Gay, M.D.	1916	F. W. Barrows, M.D.	1966	George L. Collins, Jr., M.D.
1866	George Abbott, M.D.	1917	Irving W. Potter, M.D.	1967	Edward C. Rozek, M.D.
1867	Joshua R. Lothrop, M.D.	1918	George F. Cott, M.D.	1968	Guy S. Alfano, M.D.
1868	John Boardman, M.D.	1919	James E. King, M.D.	1969	James R. Nunn, M.D.
1869	Orlando K. Parker, M.D.	1920	Earl P. Lothrop, M.D.	1970	Charles D. Bauer, M.D.
1870	Julius F. Miner, M.D.	1921	Arthur G. Bennett, M.D.	1971	Anthony P. Santomauro, M.D.
1871	William Gould, M.D.				

Shown here are the names of the past presidents of the Medical Society of the County of Erie for the years 1821–1971.

Past Presidents
Medical Society of Erie County

1972	Leonard Berman, MD	1997	Franklin Zeplowitz, MD
1973	James H. Cosgriff, Jr., MD	1998	Nedra J. Harrison, MD
1974	Frank J. Bolgan, MD	1999	Datta C. Wagle, MD
1975	Ralph J. Argen, MD	2000	Ross L. Guarino, MD
1976	Carmelo S. Armenia, MD	2001	Susan Baldassari, MD
1977	Anthony J. Federico, MD	2002	Donald P. Copley, MD
1978	John J. Giardino, MD	2003	Richard J. Buckley, MD
1979	George W. Fugitt, MD	2004	Kenneth H. Eckhert, Jr., MD
1980	Joseph A. Prezio, MD	2005	Richard P. Vienne, DO
1981	Milford Maloney, MD	2006	Philip J. Aliotta, MD
1982	Edmond J. Gicewicz, MD	2007	Ernesto Diaz-Ordaz, MD
1983	James F. Phillips, MD	2008	Edward K. Bartels, MD
1984	Victorino Anllo, MD	2009	Kathleen T. Grimm, MD
1985	Leo E. Manning, MD	2010	Eugene Kalmuk, Jr., MD
1986	Allen L. Lesswing, MD	2011	Mark J. Lema, MD
1987	Thomas W. Bradley, MD	2012	Raymond V. Paolini, Jr., MD
1988	W. Luther Musselman, MD	2013	Thomas Lombardo, Jr., MD
1989	Nancy H. Nielsen, MD, PhD	2014	John B. Wiles, MD
1990	William K. Major., Jr., MD	2015	Charles E. Wiles, III, MD
1991	Amy H. Early, MD	2016	Timothy F. Gabryel, MD
1992	H. John Rubinstein, MD	2017	Willie Underwood III, MD, MPH
1993	Richard M. Peer, MD	2018	John A. Gillespie, MD
1994	David O. Scamurra, MD	2019	Kenneth Eckhert III, MD
1995	Irene Snow, MD	2020	Stanley Pietrak, MD
1996	Russell W. Bessette, DDS, MD		

2021 Robert Armstrong, MD

Pictured here are the names of the past presidents of the Medical Society of the County of Erie for the years 1972 to 2021.

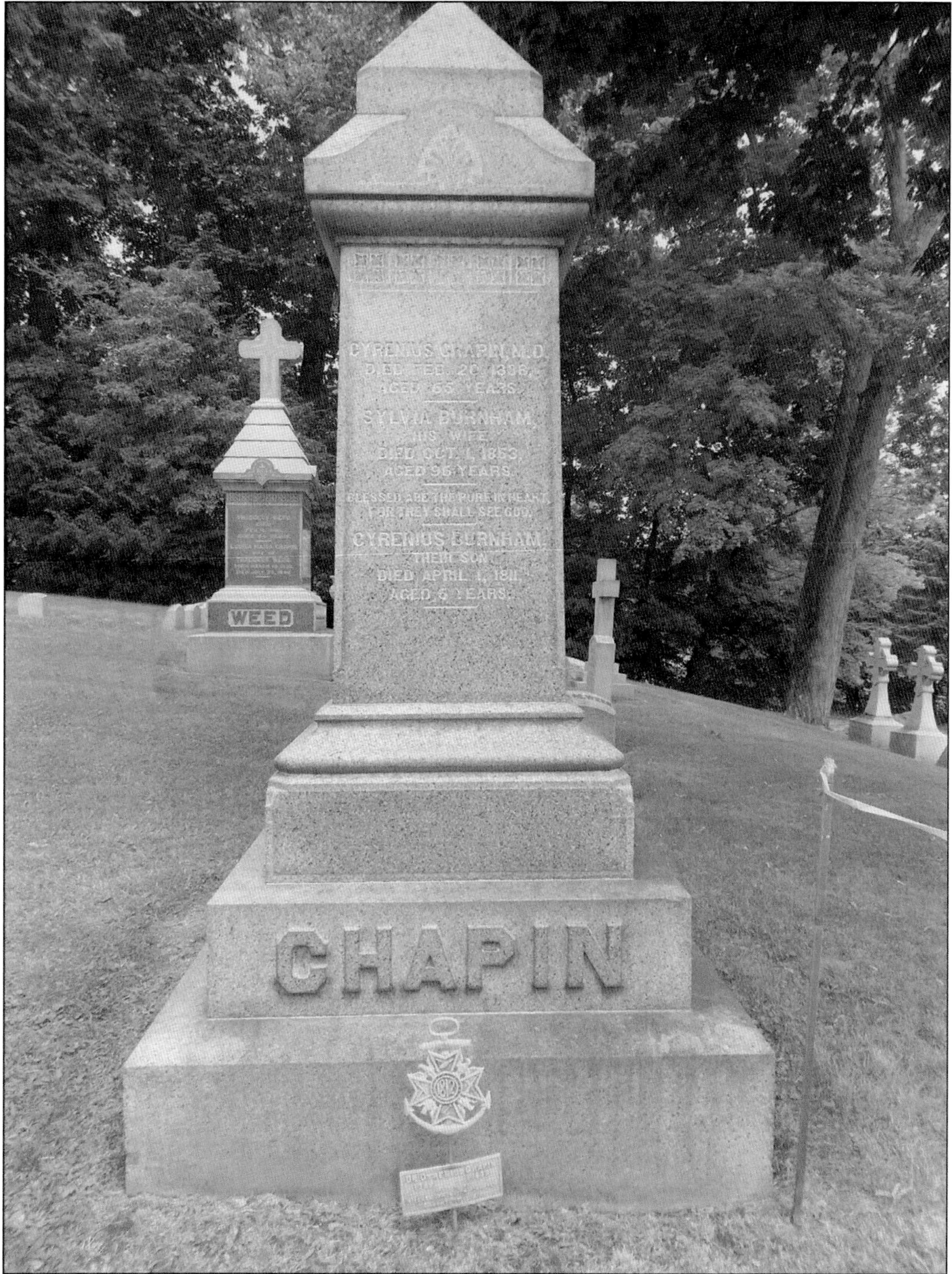

This is the gravestone of Medical Society founder and first president Cyrenius Chapin, who was captured by the British while serving as a major in the War of 1812. Following his release, Dr. Chapin returned to Buffalo and held the first Medical Society of Erie County meeting on September 1, 1821. He was laid to rest in Forest Lawn Cemetery in downtown Buffalo.

Consistent with our mission to preserve history on a local level, this book was printed in South Carolina on American-made paper and manufactured entirely in the United States. Products carrying the accredited Forest Stewardship Council (FSC) label are printed on 100 percent FSC-certified paper.

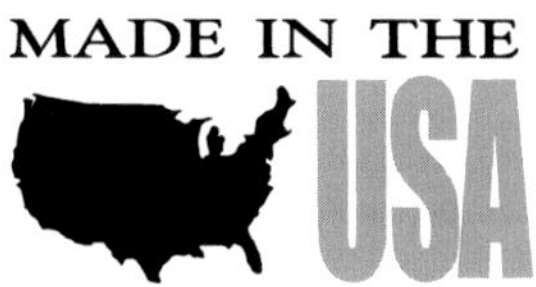